A Dream
IMPOSSIBLE!

Brian S. Langton's

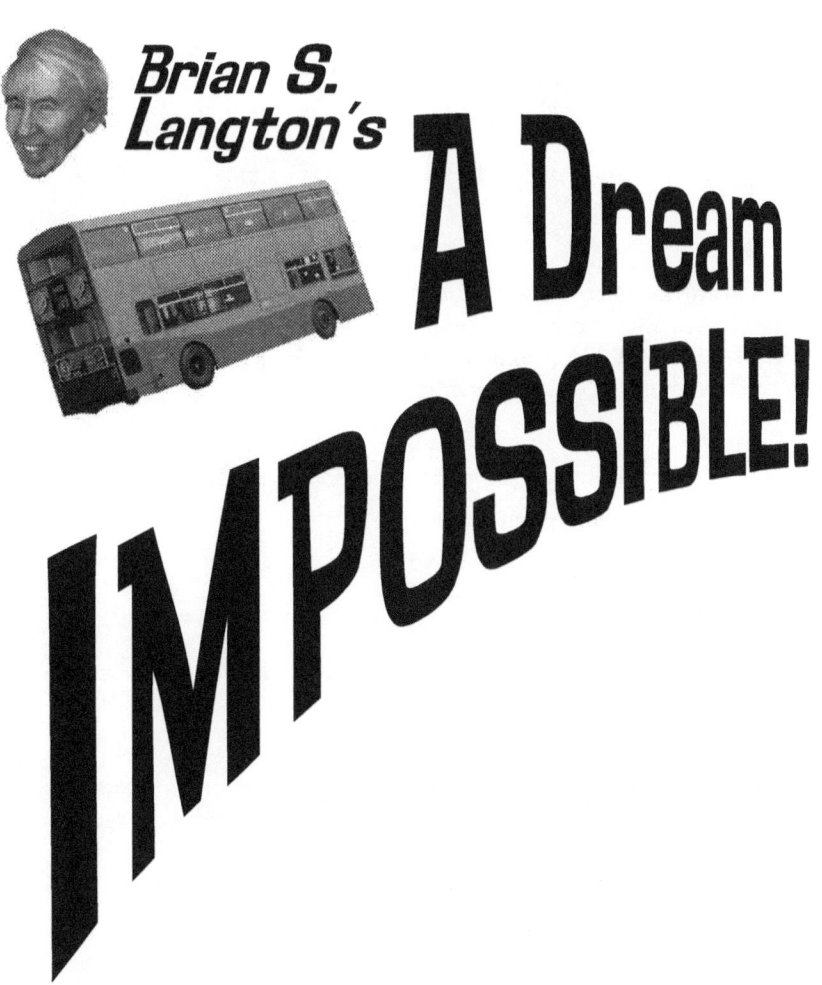

A Dream IMPOSSIBLE!

The Exciting Dream Adventures of a Guillain-Barre Syndrome Patient!

Contact the author in care of Trafford Publishing: Suite 6E, 2333 Government St., Victoria, B.C., Canada V8T 4P4. Phone: 250-383-6864 Toll-free: 1-866-638-6884 (Canada & US) Fax: 250-383-6814 E-mail: sales@trafford.com Web site: www.trafford.com

Cover and Interior Book Design by Pneuma Books, LLC

For more info, visit www. pneumabooks.com

Note for Librarians: a cataloguing record for this book that includes Dewey Classification and US Library of Congress numbers is available from the National Library of Canada. The complete cataloguing record can be obtained from the National Library's online database at: www.nlc-bnc.ca/amicus/index-e.html

ISBN 1-4120-1064-0

TRAFFORD

This book was published on-demand in cooperation with Trafford Publishing.
On-demand publishing is a unique process and service of making a book available for retail sale to the public taking advantage of on-demand manufacturing and Internet marketing. On-demand publishing includes promotions, retail sales, manufacturing, order fulfilment, accounting and collecting royalties on behalf of the author.

Suite 6E, 2333 Government St., Victoria, B.C. V8T 4P4, CANADA
Phone   250-383-6864   Toll-free   1-888-232-4444 (Canada & US)
Fax   250-383-6804   E-mail   sales@trafford.com
Web site www.trafford.com   TRAFFORD PUBLISHING IS A DIVISION OF TRAFFORD HOLDINGS LTD.
Trafford Catalogue #03-1433   www.trafford.com/robots/03-1433.html
10   9   8   7   6   5   4   3   2

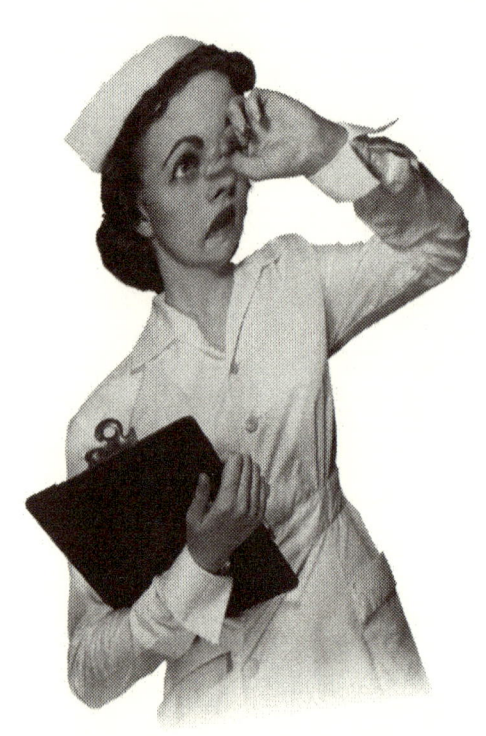

Table of Contents

Author's Preface ix

A Comic Figure 1
GBS Patient on a Secret Mission 5
Ottawa Summers 39
Wild Dogs Attack 47
The Debt Collector 57
Flying Bombs 61
Submariner in Trouble 65
Downtown Adventures 69
Jet Fighters on Call 79
Catastrophe 83
Precious Stone 95
Quicksand Floor 101
Sheriff's Office 109
Guardian Angel in a Stetson 115
Part-Time Patient 123
Heavy Snowfall Warning 131
Daylight Robbery 141
Who Wants to Buy a Double Decker Bus 149
Across the Great Lake 159

Author Acknowledgements 165

About the Author 167

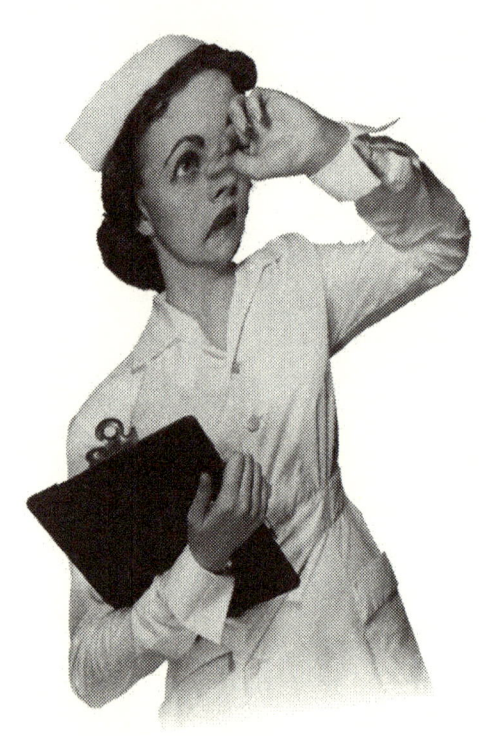

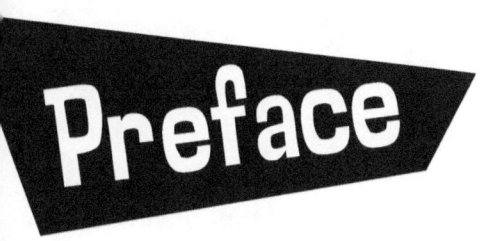

Preface

After I had published my first book, A First Step—Understanding Guillain-Barré Syndrome, it occurred to me that the Dream Sequences described in that book would make for interesting reading on their own, as a collection of short – but impossible – stories.

Thus were sown the seeds for this publication. The 'postscripts' that have been added are included to assist readers who have not read the earlier book, and who therefore may not having a full understanding of the circumstances in which I found myself.

During my seven-month confinement in Intensive Care, on a ventilator for breathing assistance, diagnosed with severe acute chronic Guillain-Barré Syndrome – sometimes referred to in its abbreviated form as GBS – I experienced many dreams and hallucinations, some of which are described here. The medications I was taking, the inability to distinguish between night and day, being thrust into an unfamiliar environment, or something inherent in the disease itself may have been the cause. Although these dreams are not necessarily in the sequence in which I dreamed them, it is possible to connect them to certain events or phases of my illness.

Initially, I was paralysed from my toes up to my eyebrows. This did not appear to inhibit my mobility in some of the dreams though. One moment I was in a wheelchair, the next flying an F16 fighter jet, even though I had never flown before, other than as a fare paying passenger.

I found these episodes much more intense than the garden-variety dream. In fact, most seemed so real that sometimes it was difficult, if not impossible, to separate them from reality. Every effort has been made to keep to the original story lines. It must, of course, be understood there were a few—although very few—grey areas, and only in those situations have I linked different parts of the story by the logical threads suggested by circumstances. For the most part, my recall of these dreams was total.

Except for my relatives, the names used to identify characters are fictitious and used to enable the reader to follow the thread of the story. In these sequences, any similarity to any person, living or deceased, other than in the case of the exception noted, is entirely coincidental and unintended.

I hope you enjoy your read.

~ Author

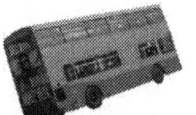

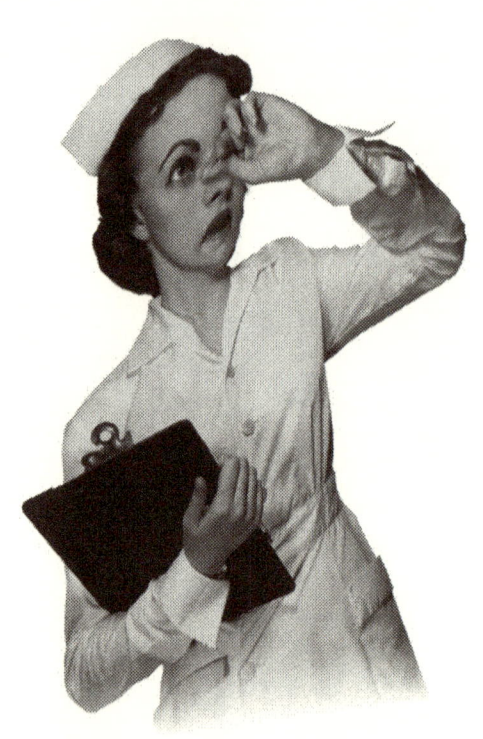

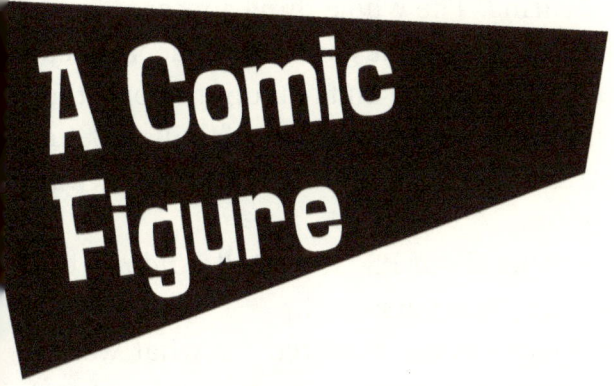

A Comic Figure

I was convinced that the reason a neck brace was put on me every time I was transferred from my hospital bed to a wheelchair was to make me look foolish. I imagined it gave me the likeness of an English comic figure, Billy Bunter. Billy was, as I recall, a very plump and greedy fellow with ugly, fat protruding lips accentuated by sunken cheeks. That is exactly how the brace made me feel.

The brace had two parts with an opening in the front of the bottom half for connections to the ventilator or the oxygen supply. The connection had to be changed whenever I was taken farther away from the ventilator than the cable would allow. I was, naturally, more conscious of wearing it when I was out of my room, and that made me suspicious of the motives of anyone suggesting such an outing.

If it were a publicity stunt, a significant number of people must have been involved, I figured, because it took six or seven nurses to get me out of bed and into the chair. I was sure they were not all involved, though, since most of them were very kind and caring. The whole thing appeared to me to be the work of the director of the government department that was interested in publicizing and obtaining support for Guillain Barre Syndrome patients and their families, better known as the department of PS-GBS-PAF. The trouble was, I could not identify him.

I did not like anything about PS-GBS-PAF! I did not like the way they worked or their personnel.

One afternoon I recall being prepared for what was to become a familiar outing. On went my brace and I endured the transfer to the wheelchair. I knew I was surrounded by friends, yet I was equally sure there was at least one person from the 'department' in their midst.

It was a beautiful sunny day, and so warm and comfortable that, except for the brace, I was starting to forget about all my suspicions. Not for long though. Suddenly I was flooded with the knowledge that something was being planned for me. I was to be enlisted on a secret mission.

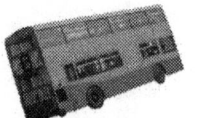

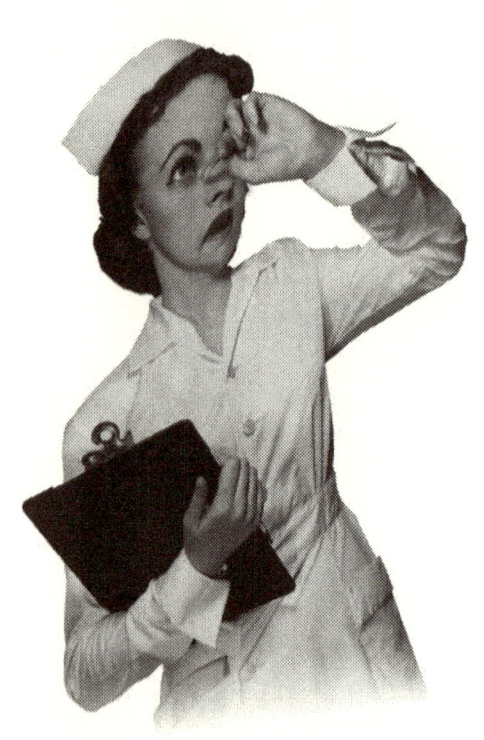

GBS Patient on a Secret Mission

I was enjoying the spacious surroundings at our weekend cottage in Calgary. It was on a lot in a very quiet subdivision, and its back garden bordered the land occupied by the Hotel Deluxe. The funny thing was, I could only vaguely remember how to get there.

The hotel itself was a fine piece of architecture ten stories high, with the usual swimming pool between the rear of the hotel and my property. It was good to have a pleasant area next door.

As I was relaxing in the cottage garden on this particular day, I could see a group of three people—two very smartly dressed businessmen and a very attractive young blonde woman, whom I assumed to be a sales person—at one of the hotel's umbrella-covered tables. They were looking and pointing in my direction, as though I were the subject of their conversation. I thought I recognized one of the men as the director of a government department interested in publicizing and obtaining support for Guillain-Barré Syndrome patients and their families.

It became very clear that I was the topic of their conversation when the three of them got up and started walking towards the gateway that separated the hotel from my cottage. I beckoned them to come through to join me.

I now knew I had correctly identified one of the men as Manny Olafson, the director. He had once provided tickets for my wife, Sylvia and me to go on two short vacations as part of the healing process. He had then turned around and used me for his own publicity purposes, which made me feel very foolish because I was displayed in a tight-fitting neck brace. I did not want to be used in such a distasteful way again.

The three came over to where I was sitting, and the person I recognized as Manny introduced me to his colleagues Tommy Tomlinson and Grizelda Fredericks. As I expected, Manny offered me another trip, but this time it did not include Sylvia. He refused to name the destination, but suggested I would enjoy the time away from the hospital. Remembering the last two trips and believing the purpose was again a publicity stunt, I refused.

Manny, however, would not take no for an answer. He used every argument he could think of to try to persuade me to accept his offer. Finally, he could see he was getting nowhere and got up to leave. Tommy and Grizelda left with him.

Now, I thought to myself, *I can relax and enjoy the sun with the knowledge that I do not have to put up with anymore of Manny's distasteful publicity trips.* Little did I know that they were not about to let the matter drop. This became clear when Grizelda appeared again at my gate. I had no alternative but to invite her to join me. She continued pressing me to accept the trip that Manny was offering, arguing that in view of everything that he and his colleagues were trying to do for me and fellow Guillain-Barré sufferers, I should have the decency to at least consider his offer. She reminded me that they were solely interested in raising funds to improve awareness, treatments, and research.

Again I said no, and Grizelda could see that I was adamant. Indeed I was. If Sylvia wasn't included, there was no way I would accept. At this point, Grizelda's demeanour changed. "What if I can persuade Manny and the department to include Sylvia? Would that make a difference?" she asked.

I thought for a few moments and, with a feeling that I might live to regret my decision, agreed to go. I told her it would also be nice to know where we would be going. I was a little concerned about the secrecy and wondered why it was necessary.

She left to talk to Manny and, maybe an hour later, returned with confirmation that the department had agreed to allow both Sylvia and me to go on the trip. She could not, however, let me know the destination.

The next morning, just as I was about to enjoy my coffee in the garden, who should appear but Manny looking very pleased with himself. "I'm glad you have agreed to go on the trip, but please, mention this to no one. You will understand why later," he said. Still puzzled by the secrecy, I reluctantly agreed. By this time I was starting to suspect I was dealing with the government. Again, I asked about the destination, but all Manny would say was that I shouldn't worry and I would be advised later.

I spent the next few days relaxing, although the forthcoming trip was on my mind and I was making sure we would be ready to leave on short notice.

Then one morning Tommy Tomlinson arrived with one of his colleagues, a man named Peter Woodward, whom I'd not met before. "Okay, let's go," said Tommy. "Everything has been arranged. We have your tickets here, and Sylvia's will be delivered to her separately since she will be meeting up with you later."

With that, we were off to Southport Road in Calgary. For readers not familiar with Calgary, Southport Road is a narrow street bordered by trees and an arterial roadway on one side and buildings of perhaps eight stories on the other. When we got there, a shining new Boeing 737 was waiting. Tommy and Peter helped me board the plane, which was full. This surprised me since it was supposed to be a top-secret mission. Tommy assessed the situation and told Peter to go to the tail section and try to make room for an extra seat. I'm not sure how he accomplished this, but somehow he managed. With me rather awkwardly seated between Tommy and Peter who were standing, Tommy signalled that we were ready for take-off.

I had experienced some white-knuckled take-offs, but none like this one. With the engines roaring and Tommy and Peter holding me in my seat, the plane was in the air. Or was it? We seemed to climb a bit, but then dove and levelled out with the office buildings at eye level. Then we climbed again, and the captain came over the intercom and apologized, saying the rough take-off was caused, no doubt, by the extra seat in the back!

"Okay, where are we headed and where is Sylvia?" I asked Tommy.

"Don't worry. Sylvia will be meeting up with us later. I am only cleared to tell you that we will be landing at Red Deer International Airport," he answered. (For those not familiar with Red Deer, Alberta, there is no international airport anywhere close.) "All the passengers are obviously aware that we are flying into Red Deer," Tommy went on, "so there was no secret about this part of the journey. I will let you know our ultimate destination when we take off on the next leg."

The landing at Red Deer was a little bumpy, but otherwise uneventful. After the other passengers had disembarked, I was led into the airport building. Peter said we should go to one of the offices in the customs area and he would then explain the purpose of the trip and provide me with some important information. Tommy added that Manny would meet us there. One of the customs officers recognized Tommy and pointed to one of the offices, indicating that we would not be disturbed.

When we got to the room, Manny was there, along with another familiar-looking person who had the sort of face that you see on television many times but cannot put a name to. Manny welcomed me, said he hoped I'd had a good flight to Red Deer, and introduced the other man as Minister of the Department of Foreign Affairs and International Trade. The minister shook my hand warmly and said he hoped I would be up to the mission they had in mind for me.

"Mission?" I asked, "You said *mission*, not trip."

The minister looked a little embarrassed and said that the nature of the journey had not been disclosed for security reasons. He apologized and gestured us to sit down at a large table.

"Even now," said the minister, "I am unable to tell you the exact destination; but you are headed for a developing country and will be part of a very secret mission—so secret, in fact, that before leaving you will be required to sign a waiver signifying that you will not admit to having any connection with this country and that you will defend the government against any claim for any reason whatsoever. "Also," he went on, "I have to tell you that, should you be captured and taken prisoner, the government will deny any knowledge of you. The purpose of the mission is twofold— to support freedom fighters fighting for democracy and to create greater awareness of the Guillain-Barré Syndrome, which does not distinguish between people. As we all know, G.B.S. is a very rare condition. You are one of the few people currently afflicted, and you were chosen because you are capable of supporting a better understanding of Guillain-Barré. This is a politically sensitive area, and the utmost security must be observed. We are aware of at least one foreign power that, to put it mildly, would take great exception to our presence in that part of the world. What do you think, Brian?"

Dare I tell him that I felt very taken advantage of, but also thought it might be fun? It was a little like being on a roller coaster—once the thing starts, there's no getting off until the ride is over. "Look," I said, "I don't appreciate being kept in the dark, but I do understand the reasons for it. Yes, I will accept a place on the mission, providing Sylvia can join me. But I must know when she and I can meet up."

"Good," said the minister. "I will make a phone call after which I, hopefully, will have an answer for you."

Sylvia, meanwhile, was shopping with our daughter Sally. Just before they were about to return home, Sally remembered she had to make a phone call. She parked and went in search of a pay phone, leaving Sylvia alone. As soon as Sally was out of sight, two secret service agents approached, showed their identification, and asked Sylvia to accompany them. They explained that they would be taking her to join me, but for security reasons, her disappearance had to look like a kidnapping.

Sylvia protested, but her efforts were to no avail. The agents reminded her that national security and the safety of the mission were involved. With that, they quickly ushered her to a waiting sport utility vehicle and drove away.

"I have spoken to Ottawa," the minister said, turning to face me, "and understand that arrangements have been made for your wife to meet you at the top-secret overseas staging area in Okotoks, Alberta. We shall be flying there in about two hours. We did not go there directly because flights from Calgary would surely be tracked on radar by the foreign powers interested in the developing country we have tar- geted. Flights out of Red Deer will not be monitored or attract attention. For our mission to succeed, we have to ensure the utmost secrecy. In the meantime," he continued, "I must ask you to sign this waiver, which apart from freeing the government from all liability for anything which might happen to you, requires that you not carry modern medicines or anything else that would indicate that you are not a citizen of our target country."

I was particularly alarmed at the notion of being without antibiotics because I had pneumonia. The thought of having to wait until my return to North America to resume my treatment, or worse, of becoming sicker while overseas really scared me. I discussed my concern with the minister, but could see I would get nowhere. "All right," I said finally. "Pass me the documents and I will sign. I am committed to the mission and will see this through, but I'd really like to know who will be traveling with me and what relevance this mission has to publicizing the Guillain–Barre Syndrome?"

"Sure," replied the minister. "In addition to the crew, you will be accompanied by approximately forty others, including engineers, technicians, mercenaries, and a medical staff of five. There will be two doctors on the team, and it will be their responsibility to arrange for visits to hospitals and clinics when we arrive at our destination—which you will be advised of when we reach the overseas staging area in Okotoks. You and Manny will leave in about an hour. Sylvia and the others will be arriving there independently. I hope this answers your questions."

"Fine," I said. "That is good to know."

In less than an hour, Manny and I were on an old DC3 for the forty-five minute flight to Okotoks.

Our landing was uneventful, considering the age of the plane. As we disembarked, I thanked the pilot; then we proceeded to a building in the staging area. Security was very tight. I said goodbye to Manny and was ushered by an agent of some kind through a maze of corridors to an office in a large hangar-type building, where I was asked to wait. After about ten minutes, a nurse came in and told me I was going to be given a medical examination and checked out for any modern drugs or antibiotics that may have been in my system. She said that I shouldn't worry; I would be made comfortable.

At this point, two men came into the office. "Hello, I guess you are Brian," said one. "My name is Alan, and I would like to introduce you to Lieutenant Colonel Randolph Hillier, the commanding officer of the staging unit."

"Hi Brian, I am pleased to meet you," said the lieutenant colonel, "Please call me Randy. I know are wondering where we will be sending you. Your destination is Boravia, and you will be accompanied by a number of dedicated professionals, including the medical people with whom you will be working—if everything goes well, that is. Do you have any questions?"

"Yes I do have questions. I presume the mercenaries with whom I am traveling will be responsible for our security en route, but what happens once we land in Boravia? Will we be on our own?"

"Pretty much," Randy admitted. "That's why when you get there, it will be important to blend into the local community as well as you can, avoiding, where possible, any connection to our country. We cannot appear to be sending

13

in an independent security force. You will be visiting several hospitals and clinics with the medical team, but, as for the mercenaries, they have other business."

I told Randy I understood, at which point he said he would leave me for now so I could proceed with my medical exam.

As he and Alan left the office, the nurse reappeared and called for an assistant to bring in a stretcher. Some stretcher! It was more like a trestle table on wheels. At least it had a thin mattress to make the surface a little more bearable. I was helped—or more accurately, lifted—onto the table and left while the nurse went to prepare the equipment necessary for my exam.

As I would have expected, it was at least half an hour before she returned. In the meantime, Alan came in and told me he had an invitation for me from the chief. "There will be an F-16 fighter jet on the airfield tomorrow morning, and he wonders if you would like to fly it."

"You bet I would," I replied.

"Flown before?" Alan asked.

"Only as a fare-paying passenger. But I would be happy to give it a try."

Alan then explained that the F-16 would be available at 10:15 a.m. and that the wing commander would give me a run through of the flight controls. He added that he would come for me about 7:30, allowing enough time for him to help me into my flying gear.

All this time the nurse had been standing by, not sure whether to laugh or cry!

Now I was in her hands. As she started on my medical, I

14

mentioned that I felt my pneumonia was getting worse and questioned her about my prospects if I were unable to continue taking antibiotics. Her response was that old-fashioned remedies had been available before antibiotics and that appropriate ones would be issued to me. Surprisingly, this satisfied me.

At about ten the next morning, complete with my helmet, oxygen kit, ejector harness (which I had struggled with), and the rest of my flight gear, I made my way onto the airstrip and noticed an older Boeing 757 sitting at the edge of the runway. Its paint was worn away, and it looked somewhat worse for the wear. I hope we're not flying to Boravia in that, I thought. Then I saw the F-16. It was either fresh from the factory or newly painted. The wing commander had just arrived, and when he saw me, he came over to give me a cheery welcome to his wing, which consisted of three F-16's.

"Okay, let's get on-board," he said, "and I'll show you the controls. It all looks terribly complicated, but I enjoy flying these birds and think you will, too. Just think. If you bring your F-16 back safely, you will probably go on record as the oldest pilot to fly one!" I smiled at this and then began paying very serious attention to everything he was showing me in the cockpit.

The 'flying lesson' completed, the wing commander suggested I make myself comfortable behind the controls, keep my hands clear of the canopy as it closed, go through the pre-flight checks, and prepare for takeoff. The tower gave me permission to head to the main runway as soon as I was ready.

Taxiing to the designated runway was not too difficult,

and the experience gave me quite a bit of confidence, most of it probably false. I just had to make sure the F-16 did not get away from me and soon learned to apply just enough of the brake to keep her in check. Boy, this is not so bad, I thought.

I soon mastered changing directions and turning. Learning as I went, I reached the runway and radioed the tower for permission to take off, which I was promptly given. There was no other traffic in the area. Now came the big test.

I allowed the 'big bird' to start rolling forward. Gradually at first, then suddenly, tremendous 'g' forces were pressing me into the back of my seat. This was exhilarating. I increased power and was soon hurtling down the runway. Then, after gently easing back on the stick, I was airborne.

After successfully flying around the area for about half an hour, I decided to bring the aircraft back to its base and hoped I hadn't forgotten all I needed to know to land her safely. It was now white-knuckle time, as the runway appeared a lot closer than it should have been. Was it my speed or just the fact that I was not thinking quickly enough? I decided to go around one more time. I gently lifted the nose and added more power. Again the F-16 responded much faster than I expected. I was starting to sweat.

This is it—the best approach I can make, I tried to convince myself. It was like being at the top of a hill on a bicycle without any brakes. Gently I eased the craft around, feeling it was controlling me rather than the other way around. I persevered, however, and lined up with the runway, then cut back on the power and eased the plane down—if it's possible to ease down something that's travelling in excess of two hundred kilometres per hour. Closer and closer the runway appeared to be rushing towards me. I braced myself, fought to keep the F-16 from drifting to the left, and straightened up just in time to make a heavy two-point landing. Okay, so it was not a perfect touchdown. At least I made terra firma in one piece and succeeded in stopping just short of the end of the runway. Any spectators— and I'm thinking here of the wing commander in particular —must have been scared out of their wits!

On firm ground again, it was now time to return to the maintenance hangar and continue with my medical exam. I found myself back on to one of those uncomfortable stretchers and was quickly wheeled into another room, where I noticed a number of other people on similar stretchers, also seemingly preparing for their medicals. Then suddenly on the other side of the room, leaning up from her stretcher was Sylvia! She was waving madly to attract my attention. I had really mixed feelings. Don't get me wrong, it was great to see her there, but what had I got her into? No wonder "the department" and their spokesman Manny had resisted including her. At least I have to give them credit for keeping their word. "See you soon!" I called to her.

At this point, the nurse took control and put me through some gruelling tests. As she took a blood pressure reading, she mentioned having seen me land. "Enough," I said. "Let's not talk about that. It wasn't the best part of the flight!" She smiled without saying anything and continued with her work. While this was happening I could see that Sylvia was also getting medical work done.

The next morning the medical team, Sylvia, and I were given a briefing on the conditions we were likely to encounter at our destination, which we now knew to be Boravia. Since we had to avoid immigration and customs, we would not be landing at the capital. In all probability, the landing was going to be a rough one, but our agents in the field had assured us that the runway would be just long enough for our 757. While this was going on, we could hear jet engines being powered up.

We were going to have to live pretty primitively, but at least the temperature would be in the thirties (Centigrade). Captain Rob Jefferson, the briefing officer, asserted, "The nearest town or village is deep in the bush, some forty kilometres from our runway. A driver, who will have a Bedford truck at his disposal, will meet us; and from there, we will be making for Newport, the capital. To avoid any suspicion as to our identities, we are going to have to make it look as though we are simply entering the capital from within the country." With that, he wrapped up the meeting and asked us to be ready to board in two hours. "I will be with you as part of the medical team, so if there are any more questions we can address them on the flight."

After a farewell dinner in the mess hall, those of us who were departing for Boravia assembled in front of the main hangar and started to make our way towards a parked Boeing 757, freshly painted in Boravian Air colours. The forty or fifty people ready to board would certainly not fill the aircraft, but as we later discovered, a large number of seats had been removed for cargo and supplies. Once onboard, Sylvia and I chose our seats—not in my favourite window position—and started to make ourselves comfortable. I could not help noticing that the condition inside the aircraft did not match the fresh paint on the outside, and the few seats were cramped and well worn. The interior design was from another age. It reminded me of the sixties! All around people were smoking, and I remember hoping that a "Please extinguish all cigarettes" sign would appear before takeoff.

The moment of truth had arrived. The jet's engines were revving up loudly now, and on came the signs—not only "Fasten seat belts," but also "Please extinguish all cigarettes." So far, so good. We started to taxi towards the runway.

Speaking as though we were all fare-paying passengers, the captain came on the intercom, welcomed us, and thanked us for choosing to fly Boravian Air. As he was drawing attention to the 'Fasten seat belts sign', his demeanour changed, and he suddenly exclaimed, "What idiot left an F-16 on the end of the runway?" I wished I were an ostrich and could have stuck my head in the sand to avoid my embarrassment.

The pilot must have had clearance, since the engines appeared to be almost at full power, and then we started to roll. All conversations ceased as we accelerated down the runway. A gentle bump, then a harder one, and we were airborne. I guess in the interim, some kind person must have moved the F-16!

We seemed to be climbing for a long time. The quiet that settled in during take off remained for some time. There was a good deal of turbulence, and it was really bumpy until we appeared to be at cruising altitude. Then normal conversations and joking around resumed.

Our flight, which from that point was uneventful, seemed to go on forever. I did not time it, but after what seemed like seven or eight hours, the captain announced that we were about to descend and that all normal formalities, including the fastening of seatbelts, should be observed. "The crew hopes you enjoyed your flight with Boravian Air and that you will fly with us again," crooned the captain's voice over the intercom. Except for a little more turbulence, our landing was fairly routine until we actually touched down. At that point the ride became quite rough. When we finally came to a standstill, we started to relax and congratulate each other on still being in one piece.

Rob Jefferson came over to where Sylvia and I were seated and explained that we would be exiting the aircraft with the medical team, including him, and leaving the others behind for their top-secret briefing. I do not have a clear recollection of how we disembarked. There was only a clearing in the bush, a single runway with no airport or other facilities in view. Who knows? Maybe we grabbed onto a tree and shimmied down to the ground. I rather suspect, though, that some form of ladder must have been deployed from the aircraft.

The group of us, consisting of Rob, two medical doctors, two medics, Sylvia and me, were by now standing just off the runway looking for any sign of the Bedford truck that should have been sent out to meet us. There was no vehicle to be seen. We decided that, for security reasons, the driver must have gone to some pains to keep the vehicle out of sight. If he did not come out of the bushes to meet us soon, we would have to go search for him.

To the west of the airstrip there was nothing but low scrub for some distance. No place for a truck there. The east side was a different story. It was a jungle with only two apparent clearings. The one immediately opposite us was the obvious first choice to head into to look for our driver.

It wasn't long before we spotted what we were looking for. There was the Bedford. Although it appeared some effort had been made to hide it at the side of the clearing, it didn't take us long to find it. But where was the driver? There was something odd here.

Rob and I went for a closer look. What we saw horrified us. When we opened the passenger-side door, there was a figure slumped over the steering wheel, his head covered in blood. One of the medics had joined us by now, and he felt for a pulse. There was none. After further checks, the medic turned to us and indicated something we did not wish to hear—the driver had been dead for some time.

Now what? Here we were, miles from Newport confronting this grizzly death. Rob asked one of the doctors if he would drive. His name was Jock, and he was as Scottish as the misty highlands of that great country. "Of course," he replied without any hesitation. "Just give me the directions, laddy. I'll get you to Newport."

That being decided, we started to come to grips with the reality of our situation. We had to get our luggage off the plane, but first we had to give the unfortunate driver some sort of a burial. That took time, but we finally accomplished the sad task. Then it was back to the runway and the 757. We were in luck. The crew, and maybe others on the aircraft, had unloaded our equipment and supplies. Everything we needed was neatly stacked on the side of the runway. There was no activity, so we assumed the briefing was still ongoing on the plane. Jock drove up in the Bedford, and we started to load.

As soon as everything had been placed on board, we all climbed into the truck. Sylvia sat in the cab with Jock, while the rest of us made ourselves as comfortable as we could in the back amongst our boxes of equipment. Jock, looking very confident behind the wheel, turned to see if everyone was safely accommodated. A vocal chorus of "O-Kay lets go" from the five of us in the back was enough for him.

"Hold it," Rob called out to Jock. He was having second thoughts about Sylvia being up front and pointed out that her presence there could attract attention we did not need. Sylvia quickly agreed to abandon the comparative luxury of the cab and joined us in the back of the truck. Then we were off.

We drove slowly through the cleared area, which got increasingly narrow as we proceeded away from the airstrip. It was a rough ride and dusty too. This must have been their dry season.

Soon we came to another road, which could certainly not be called a main road, although it obviously carried more traffic than the one we were on. After a brief pause at the junction, we headed north towards Newport. The sun was getting lower in the sky and throwing shadows across our path. Suddenly, upon rounding a bend, we saw a roadblock. Two trucks were parked together, making passage through impossible. Standing around the barricade formed by these trucks were, perhaps, a dozen men. They appeared to be soldiers, and all brandished automatic weapons. Jock glanced quickly at Rob as if looking for directions on how to react, although he later admitted there was no option but to stop and hope we would be allowed through.

As we slowed and came to a halt just short of the barricade, the soldiers cautiously approached with their guns at the ready. The leader appeared to be a junior officer, and it was he who approached Jock and asked for I.D. One of the soldiers leapt on to the back of the Bedford, while the others encircled us. We anxiously awaited some indication as to whether we would be allowed to proceed. To our dismay, the soldier pointed his gun at each of us in turn and made it clear that he wanted our watches and any other valuables we may have had with us.

We had no alternative but to comply. Meanwhile, Jock was doing his best to convince the young officer that we had been transferring patients from Newport to the St. Augustine Auxiliary Hospital. He later said he'd recalled hearing that place name at one of his briefing sessions. The officer had obviously noticed the blood on the dashboard and lower section of the windshield, and Jock hoped his story would sound convincing.

"What sort of patients?" questioned the officer?

"Bleeders," Jock replied, and the soldier seemed satisfied. In the meantime, things were not going so well in the back. We were being relieved of anything the soldiers considered of value. Not quietly though. Everyone was complaining loudly, and that made our adversaries very nervous. By then, another two had climbed in and were helping to collect the loot.

Due to the noise we were making, no one noticed a northbound vehicle rounding the bend in the road behind us. Its headlights were off and it approached quietly and deliberately, pulling up a short distance behind us.

Suddenly, all hell broke loose. Our adversaries, so greedily involved in their hunt for instant wealth, found themselves surrounded by a large number of well-armed mercenaries, some of whom just happened to be our flight companions. The soldiers who had stopped us fired a few shots in panic and surprise at having the tables turned on them, then quickly saw they were outgunned and outnumbered. They handed our belongings back and grimly climbed down from the truck, where, following the lead of their commanding officer, they surrendered to the mercenaries. All of their weapons were confiscated and placed on the truck behind us. Round one to us.

A half dozen of the mercenaries left to take the now frightened soldiers into the bush. We were to learn later no lasting harm came to them. They were merely taken a good distance from the road, tied up, and left to their own devices. Meanwhile, Jock and Rob got to work moving the soldier's trucks so we could pass. Both vehicles were driven off the road into the bush. We were assured that the trucks were so well hidden, even if their attackers freed themselves and reached the road, they would have trouble finding them.

We all stood around for a while, talking and expressing our thanks to the mercenaries for their timely intervention. After saying their farewells, the rag tag group took leave of us, and with wry grins, suggested we keep out of further trouble.

I suggested to Rob that we leave this area and look for somewhere to bunk down some distance away. He agreed and asked Jock to load up and continue on our heading towards Newport while he kept his eyes open for some place to drive off into the bush and set up camp for the night.

The next day dawned extremely hot and humid. We gathered our belongings and clambered aboard our trusty Bedford. Jock checked to make sure everyone and everything was secure, and we were on our way. No one said anything, but we all realized that the closer we got to Newport, the greater the danger. We got within twenty kilometres of the capital. Then the rains came.

We hastily pulled the tarp over the back of the truck to cover our belongings and ourselves and concentrated on keeping dry as we sped along. Soon we left the densely wooded bush behind. Every now and again there were clearings with shanty-type buildings, some standing on their own, some in groups.

By this time, I was feeling really sick. The hot, humid weather was making my chest condition worse. If only I could get some help at the military hospital in Newport. I was in dire need of a deep suction to drain my lungs of fluid. *How can I beat this pneumonia without antibiotics?* I wondered. Normally I hated the thought of antibiotics, but for something as serious as this they were necessary.

Even though we were now on the outskirts of the capital, the road was not in very good repair. We were really getting thrown around.

"There's the hospital," Jock called out, after rounding an almost-blind corner. It was an old, but substantial, building in a well-treed river valley. "We should make it in about five minutes," he added, driving a little faster now down the fairly steep hillside. Sylvia and the others had been discussing my condition and had decided they'd better change their original plans and get me into the military hospital as soon as possible. I was in no shape to argue.

"Okay, here's what we do," said Rob. "I've already talked it over with Jock. He'll drive us to a grocery store just this side of the hospital and drop off everyone except Brian. Then he will drive to the emergency entrance. This should not cause anyone to connect them with a vehicle containing seven people being sought by the military, if indeed the word about us is out. He will stay with Brian until he is admitted. Once he's situated, we can then visit. Is everyone happy with that? I don't think we have any other choice."

Was this the way I was supposed to be visiting clinics and hospitals in Boravia to publicize Guillain-Barre Syndrome? I wondered. As we were just about to drop him, and the other passengers, including Sylvia, at the supermarket, I put the question to Rob.

"No, not exactly", he replied, very apologetically. "Like everyone else, I'd hoped your pneumonia would have cleared up by now. Your Guillain-Barré Syndrome is more than enough for you to handle, but you know what governments are like with all the bureaucracy. They want us to push ahead, regardless."

With that, he jumped out, and Jock headed for the hospital.

The next thing I knew, I was surrounded by faces. I didn't recognize where I was, but knew it must be the military hospital. People were prodding me, lifting my arms and legs, enquiring if I could feel what they were doing, and asking a host of other questions. I hoped this would not go on for too long and that I would be able to get some treatment, if not for my Guillain-Barré, certainly for my pneumonia.

It's ironic, I found myself thinking, *Here I am in the hospital belonging to the same military that tried to rob us. We are trying to help their country, and what are they doing?*

Many hours with me fitfully dropping in and out of sleep. Then I heard a familiar voice. It was Rob. "Just relax," he said. "I am going to put you to sleep. We are going to help you and make you more comfortable." I started to thank him and ask to see Sylvia, but never finished the sentence. He had gently covered my face with a cloth soaked in ether. Sylvia explained what happened sometime later.

I could hear the unmistakable sound of jet engines. I thought I was on an aircraft, but I was in a hospital bed—or was it a stretcher? Since there was an intravenous feeding bottle hanging above my head. I decided it had to be a stretcher. One of the medics came by. "What is happening?" I asked him. "Where are we going?"

"We're on our way home," he replied.

"But," I started to protest, "we haven't finished the mission yet, have we?"

"Yes sir, we have. You've been out of it for six days. It's all finished, at least as far as the medical side is concerned. Now, we're just hoping we have enough fuel to make it home. The captain says it's touch and go. We've already jettisoned the surplus equipment, including some aircraft parts, to lighten the load."

We were now on a 'white knuckle' flight for a reason very different from the norm. It's not often a shortage of fuel is the culprit.

The next few hours were tense for everyone, and surely for no one more than the captain and his co-pilot. Very little was said. The hours passed. Rob came by to check on me. "Where are we now in relation to Canada?" I asked.

"We just passed over Churchill, Manitoba," he said thoughtfully. "Normally from Churchill, it's about two and a half hours to Calgary. I hope we can make it." I nodded my agreement.

Another hour passed, and the huge jet engines were purring smoothly. It seemed impossible that anything could go wrong now. Then the dreaded announcement came, and behind the captain's voice we could hear alarms sounding in the cockpit. We all knew what was coming.

"This is your captain speaking," he said. "There is even less fuel than our earlier calculations suggested so we're going to make an emergency landing. We have permission to land at a small airstrip which, given our present distance and altitude, we should be able to reach. It will likely be a rough landing, but we will do our best to get us out of this in

28

one piece. Everyone please be seated and fasten your seat belts. When I announce that we're on final approach, please adopt the crash-landing posture, head between your knees." So this was it.

Rob came over to me with some webbing and proceeded to tie my stretcher to the plane's framework; then he fastened me securely to the stretcher. He was working quickly, but very efficiently. The last of the engines was shutting down, and then there was nothing but wind noise. It was quiet—eerie in fact.

Having taken care of me, Rob went to his own seat, sat down, and fastened his safety belt. We could all feel the descending motion of the aircraft. Sometimes it seemed to dive more steeply than at others. Everyone understood only too well that there was no room for error.

Minutes seemed like hours as we glided down from our cruising altitude. We waited. Then suddenly the co-pilot came into the main cabin just long enough to tell us to assume the crash position. "We have no intercom, and we are on final approach." After a brief pause, he added, "Hold on. We will make it. We have to." With that he went to rejoin the crew. I could only imagine what was going on in the cockpit.

One of the medics looked out the window. "Gee, we're coming in fast," he yelled. There was not much I could do. I figured I'd be lucky to survive this on a stretcher. I remember wondering if anyone had ever survived the rush of blood from the head to the feet that happens between 150 and 200 kilometres an hour.

There were a few minutes of quiet, a loud bang, and then

nothing. I must have passed out. I had obviously survived the landing, but my head was swimming and I ached all over. I tried to get up to make sure everyone else had survived and to survey the damage. With great relief I saw Sylvia. She was all right and making herself useful bandaging Jock's leg. He had a nasty looking gash just below the knee. The cabin was a mess, but fortunately everyone seemed to be accounted for. The crew must have done a great job in getting the aircraft down. No fire had resulted, and we were able to organize ourselves and use the damaged cabin as a temporary headquarters.

Rob announced he was going to survey the airstrip and find out what facilities and equipment were available. Jock offered to join him, but had to back down when he put his full weight on his leg. Meanwhile, we raided the galley. It had been some time since our last meal.

"Good news and bad news," Rob called out as he clambered back into the cabin. "Which do you want first?" Without waiting for an answer, he continued, "The good news is there is an aircraft available for us to continue our flight; the bad news is that it's an old biplane, an Avro Tutor. There are normally no aircraft on this field. We just got lucky. The Tutor had landed for refuelling. It's only a two-seater and has a full payload already—the pilot and his passenger— so we will have to hang onto whatever we can—struts, wing supports, anything. The pilot says if you can find a handhold, he will go for take off. He promises to fly as low as he safely can. The responsibility, though, is all ours. What do you think?"

"How long we would be in the air?" I asked. The Tutor

30

can't have a very high cruising speed. I would hazard a guess it's somewhere between 100 to 120 miles an hour."

"You're probably right," said Jock. "And if that's the case, it's likely to take us about five hours to reach Calgary. Quite a long time to be exposed to the elements."

"At least the air is warm," Rob added.

Regardless of the obvious risks, and without much hesitation, everyone agreed to go for it. By this time, we all wanted to get home. I had been torn out of the webbing by the impact of landing, so now had to be lifted back onto my stretcher and then carried out of the cabin and across the field to where the Avro Tutor was parked. It looked in reasonable shape, to my novice eye, anyway.

The engine was still, although the pilot was standing by. He was, no doubt, conserving fuel for the last leg of our flight, which must have been close to the limit of the aircraft's range. We didn't need any more crash landings. I hoped he had calculated the additional weight he was to carry!

I was gently transferred from my stretcher onto the lower wing. My condition made it impossible for me to grip anything, so Jock bound me, as best he could, to the struts. Once I had been secured, Sylvia and the others found places where they could hold on. Sylvia lay on the lower port wing on the other side of the struts from me; and I saw one of the medics clamber onto the wing between Sylvia and the fuselage. The only grip he had was the leading edge of the wing, but I guess he knew what he was doing. Rob was trying to make himself comfortable on the tail section. I only hoped this bird would fly with all the 'interruptions' the presence of bodies on the flying surfaces would create.

"All right, we'll start the engine," the pilot announced as he clambered into his seat. His initial passenger, who we later learned was also acting as his navigator, was already in place. The Pilot had obviously arranged for take-off assistance, for just at this moment a late-sixties-model car pulled up alongside us, and two overall-clad men alighted. One had his eye on the chocks, while the other went straight to the propeller, and going through the usual hand start motions, commenced to swing. After four or five strong downward pulls, the engine burst into life, spluttering and backfiring a little at first, but finally settling into a steady rhythmic sound. The pilot made a quick final check of his controls and called for the chocks to be pulled.

Slowly he eased the heavily burdened biplane over the grass field toward the single runway. The old Tutor felt like it would fall apart at the next bounce. Luckily, it survived, and to everyone's relief, arrived at the opposite end of the runway from where our big jet had crash-landed.

There was no control tower here to give clearance, so everything was up to the pilot. He was obviously thinking hard about the jet he had to clear at the runway's end. Could he climb high enough in time?

After getting lined up, he taxied to a halt, then opened the throttle, and we were rolling, slowly at first, then at a speed one might expect to go on a Sunday afternoon drive. Our damaged jet was starting to look awfully close, but we continued down the runway. I could feel that we'd picked up a little bit of speed. The pilot had the throttle wide open, but we still weren't going fast enough to lift. Then, just as we passed the point of no return, it seemed we might actually gain sufficient height to clear the jet.

The pilot, with a lot of courage, waited until we were almost out of room, then pulled back on the stick and, almost without waiting to leave the hardtop, banked sharply to the left. We missed the jet by inches. We'd hardly gotten through that situation when up in front of us loomed an eight-foot fence. We were so low that it looked like we might not make it, particularly in our attitude, which the pilot quickly corrected and only just in time. Again, we missed disaster by inches.

We were gaining altitude now, but slowly. We had to hope there were no high-tension cables in our path for the next twelve miles or so. If there were, this journey could be over. The navigator should know, but if he did, he wasn't saying—not that those of us clinging to the wings would have been able to hear him if he had.

The air rushing by me was now a gale force wind. In addition to being bound to the struts, I was instinctively trying to curl my fingers around them to get a grip, but of course, it was useless. I couldn't move my hands. Even willpower could not overcome the paralysis. I did manage to give Sylvia a reassuring nudge, however. In return, she gave me a kind of a half smile, which told me she not only understood, but accepted the situation we were in. "I only hope we don't run into rain," I shouted to her.

Fortunately the weather was clear. There wasn't a cloud to be seen.

Suddenly there was a piercing scream. The medic holding on to the bottom wing near Sylvia must have lost his grip. There was nothing to stop him from sliding into the void. Our height couldn't have been more than fifteen hundred feet, but for the medic, it might as well have been fifteen thousand. We looked around, encouraging one another to hang tight. I saw Rob gripping the tail section for dear life and marvelled at the pilot's skill and the ruggedness of the biplane. I thought of Jock on the starboard side and hoped he had a good handhold.

Whether it was the warm air rising or the fact that we were one body lighter, we started to gain a little altitude. Good thing, as there were some fairly high hills in our path. At least once, the pilot had to take evasive action to avoid flying into one. It was fortunate for us all that those hills were not mountains.

I started thinking that maybe the medic whom we'd lost might be all right, after all. If he had fallen to earth as we were flying over a hilltop, he may have only dropped three or four feet, rolled over a few times and survived with nothing more than a few cuts and bruises.

For those of us still hanging on, cramps were beginning to set in. Everyone's hair was flowing straight out behind them in the wind current. Tiredness was becoming a factor. It was amazing more of us hadn't plummeted to the ground.

Hours passed. Areas of my upper body, which had previously started to show some movement, were now getting numb. Suddenly, the aircraft lifted noticeably, and I wondered if we'd lost someone else. I turned and checked for Sylvia. She was very tired, but so far all right, thank goodness. I looked behind, and Rob was still perched, albeit precariously, on the tail. It occurred to me that maybe someone on the other wing had gone to sleep and just slipped off into nothingness.

Now the Tudor was really starting to climb, and we no longer had to be concerned about high-tension cables or towers. We were flying over bald prairie, so hills were no longer in the reckoning, either. That was a distinct advantage; except we now had no hilltop to drop onto if we got tired and couldn't hang on.

In the distance, the Rocky Mountains were now visible. They were a wonderful sight because they signified we were finally reaching home territory. *Perhaps now*, I thought, *my pneumonia can be completely cleared up and the rest of my treatment or therapy continued. Hopefully the prognosis will be better.*

Suddenly there it was, Calgary International Airport. Strong Chinook winds must have been blowing because we were coming in at quite an angle, but slowly. Our air speed may have been ninety knots or so, but we were only making headway against land objects at perhaps forty to fifty miles per hour. I was thinking about our fuel supply.

Suddenly, a body came falling down from the top wing, whizzing by just in front of my head and disappearing into the void below. We must have had more passengers than we realized. No wonder the old biplane had experienced so much difficulty getting and staying airborne.

The Tudor rose up—in response to losing some weight, no doubt—and then her nose dipped into an even more steep descent, which brought us down to maybe fifty feet above the runway. Boosting the power, the pilot held us in level flight for a few moments and then gently eased the aircraft down onto the runway.

We had made it—and without losing anyone else!

Post Script: It is not surprising perhaps that I should dream of flying. I had flown on many airlines before, and during our European trip just days before being diagnosed with Guillain-Barré Syndrome. But flying an F16? I have never flown any aircraft. I am not a pilot.

~ Author

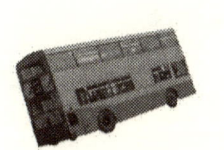

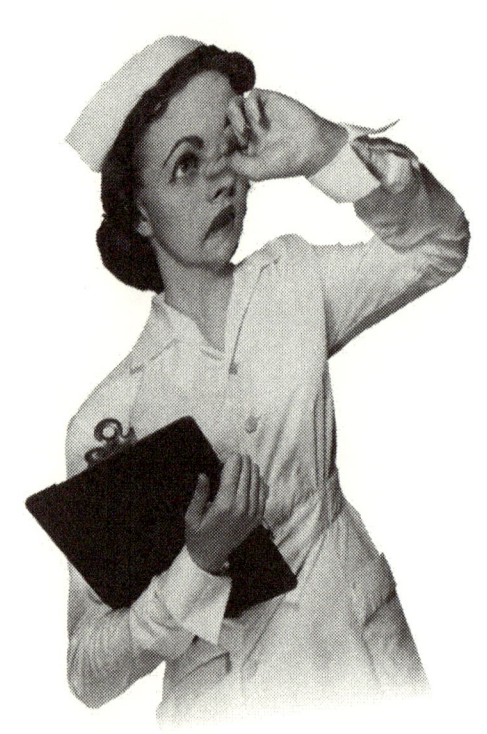

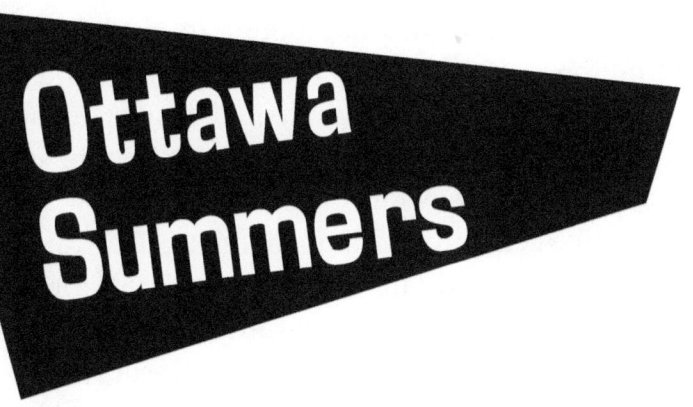

Ottawa Summers

I have no idea where this came from, but I was absolutely certain that every summer for the last few years, my wife and I had rented the Prime Minister's Ottawa home for two weeks of our vacation. Now we were going back, and this year, decided to drive instead of flying.

We arrived just in time to enjoy a beautiful sunset. As expected, we had the place to ourselves. There was a note of welcome on the table in the entrance hall, telling us which rooms were open to us; how to set the security system, which had been changed from the previous year; and giving other general information.

The arrangement was perfect. We got a free vacation, and the Prime Minister was able to vacation elsewhere, secure in the knowledge that his home was cared for.

Settling in the first night was always interesting

because remembering where everything was kept was a challenge. A lot could change in a year. When we'd found a home for all our belongings, we made ourselves a light meal. It had been a long day. I had done a lot of driving, and we'd found the change of air to be intoxicating. Those factors conspired to make us very tired, and we decided to turn in early. I followed the instructions about how to set the security system, and we went to bed.

It was a little like being in a high quality hotel. Our room was sumptuously decorated and had drapes of rich forest green velvet. The carpet was thick and lush. Through the large window we could look down on the well-lit courtyard. I could imagine the clip clopping of hooves on the cobblestones in the time before automobiles.

It took no effort at all to fall asleep. Suddenly, however, I was wide-awake and conscious of a clamour close by. Sylvia was already out of bed and putting on her housecoat. She opened the drapes about half way and called to me. I could see flashing lights. *What on earth was happening? I wondered?*

"Brian, the courtyard is flooded! There's a fire truck, pump trucks, and even the police are here." I joined her at the window just in time to see firemen turning off water sprinklers that had obviously been running for a long time. The lawns were higher than the courtyard, which was full of water.

Who had left the sprinklers on? I considered the possibility that somehow I'd punched a wrong key on the control panel when setting the security system, but that seemed unlikely. I was sure I'd followed the instructions correctly.

Maybe the head gardener or one of his people had turned the water on and forgotten it. Whatever the cause, the damage had been done, and there was nothing we could do.

After about an hour, the activity outside settled down, and eventually, there were no more flashing lights. The flooded area must have been cleaned up. Thankfully we were not disturbed. The clean-up crew probably thought the house was unoccupied.

When we awoke the next morning, it was to the sound of heavy rain. That gave us chance to look around the house and make ourselves comfortable. The view from the lounge was exceptional. The grounds were extensive, and there were some beautiful trees, many of which I knew didn't grow in our province. We decided we were really going to enjoy this holiday.

The following day dawned under a clear blue sky. Not the day to be staying in bed, we showered, dressed, enjoyed an early breakfast, and set off on a walk through the grounds and adjoining woods. We must have gone eight or nine miles. It was almost lunchtime when we returned, just in time to see a car entering the courtyard. The driver parked and waited. He appeared to be talking to a female passenger. We went into the house, deciding that whoever it was would ring the doorbell. In the meantime, we had earned a rest and some refreshment, and that was taking priority.

A short while after we'd finished eating lunch, the doorbell rang. I opened the door to a man and a woman. The fellow introduced himself as Jim and told me his wife's name was Sophie. They claimed to be relatives of the prime minister and explained that the residence had been offered to them for their sole use for the next week. I shook my head in disbelief. "My wife and I rent this residence for the same two weeks every year," I said. "There has to be some mistake. Do you have anything in writing?"

"No," Sophie claimed rather indignantly, "we are family. We don't need arrangements like this in writing."

"I think you do," I said. "We have a legal lease. On your own admission, you do not. So, how can I help you?" Realizing they were at a distinct disadvantage, Sophie backed down and became more reasonable.

"This is a large residence," she said. "Couldn't we just agree to share it for a week? Perhaps you would allow us to use the west wing?"

"Come on in," I said. "We can talk about it."

After some discussion, we came to an agreement. Sylvia and I certainly had no need of the whole house, so allowing Jim and Sophie to occupy the west wing was no hardship, except that we would have to share the lounge. Since we were expecting to be out most of the time anyway, I couldn't see that it would be a problem. The next few days passed uneventfully — that is, until the third evening.

Sylvia and I had finished supper and retired to the lounge with coffee when Sophie walked in, sat herself down, and casually asked, "Could I have a coffee? My husband has decided to make an early night of it."

"Help yourself," said Sylvia. It's in the kitchen."

That was obviously not the response she wanted, and without further comment, she stomped out of the room.

I grinned at Sylvia. "Perhaps you should have prepared

her supper, too," I said, ducking just in time to avoid one of her playful backhands.

The next day, after a pleasant time spent exploring our surroundings further, we decided to go out for supper. In spite of its challenging location on the twelfth floor, we chose a popular downtown restaurant, which was recognized for its excellent cuisine. After parking in the underground garage, we took the elevator, which for some reason didn't go any higher than the eleventh floor. We got out and followed the signs pointing the way to the twelfth floor and eventually reached a door that appeared to open to the outside of the building, allowing a panoramic view of downtown. My first reaction was to take a step back.

When we looked past the breath-taking beauty of the sparkling city lights, we saw that beyond the door there was little more than a metal landing and a narrow stairway with short treads, much like a fire escape. The only support was a very flimsy looking rail. Neither Sylvia nor I cared much for heights. We looked at each other and, without speaking, agreed that we had to overcome this scary obstacle.

As we gingerly climbed the stairs, we tried to avoid looking down. We must have been some two hundred feet above the roadway, for vehicles looked like toys and people like ants. One glance and my stomach was in my mouth. The wind at that height was quite strong, and I had a couple of bad moments. It was with much relief that we stepped onto the upper landing only to confront outward-opening doors. Stepping backwards on a small, open landing was not my idea of fun, but we'd come this far, and it was the only way in. Amazingly, we managed to keep our balance.

Our meal was excellent and exceptionally well served. We enjoyed it, in spite of the thought of having to return down the rickety staircase when we had finished.

I paid the bill and was holding Sylvia's coat for her, when I noticed the smile on the coat check girl's face. "You won't need that, sir," she remarked, pointing to the coat.

"Why not," I asked. "It's a cool night out there, and my wife will feel the chill on her way down those outside stairs."

"No, no, no. You don't go out that way!" she exclaimed. "It's only how you come in. For leaving, we have a small elevator."

We were quite relieved. That outside staircase was treacherous, and I didn't even want to think about it.

Over the next few days we continued hiking and enjoying the countryside. The warm, sunny days made us wish we could stay an extra week. That was not to be, however, and with the holiday over, it was time to load up the car and make our way home. Little did we know what terrifying experiences lay ahead, but that's another story.

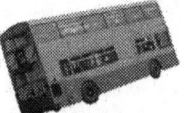

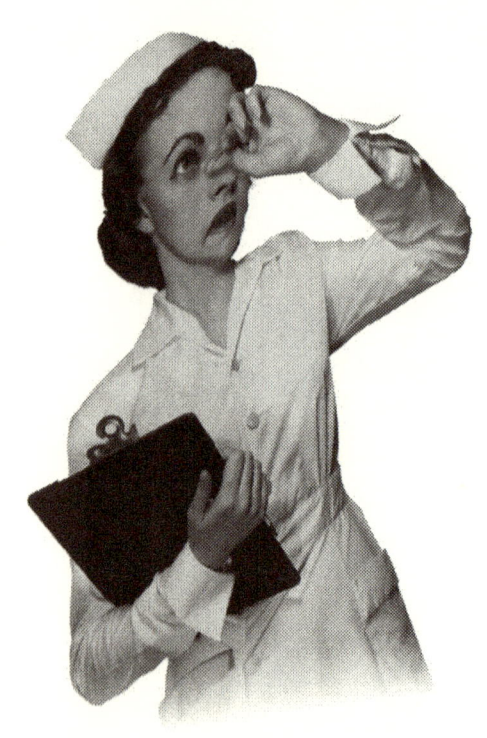

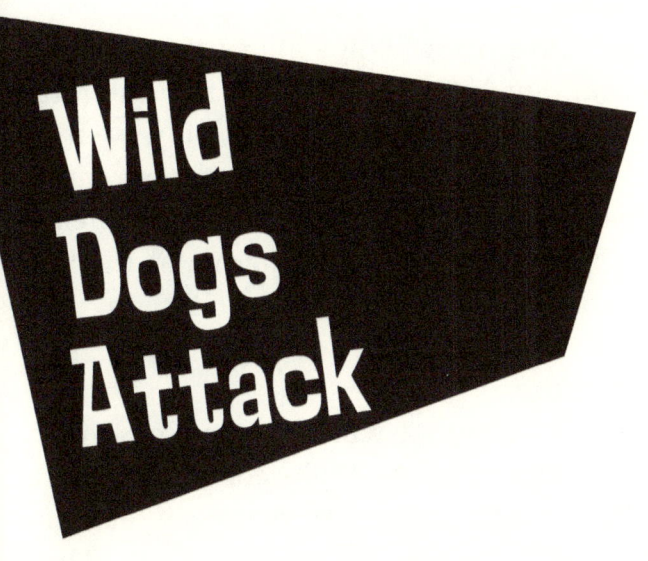

Wild Dogs Attack

We were making good progress on our drive home from Ottawa. The weather was ideal for travelling, and we were getting close to Swift Current, Saskatchewan. While driving over the prairie, both Sylvia and I had observed small off-white animals. Sometimes they were in pairs; then at other times, they'd be in larger packs. On one occasion there must have been at least a dozen of them chasing a coyote. They looked a little like dogs—and perhaps they were wild dogs, but we had only seen them at a distance, so it was difficult to tell.

Now, with the prairie and its animals behind us, we were concentrating on finding a place to gas up and have a snack. I was ready for a drink. Driving always made me thirsty, rather than hungry.

We soon came upon signs welcoming visitors to Swift

Current, population 14,000, and within minutes, came upon familiar signs advertising filling stations. Selecting one which had a restaurant alongside, I pulled into the fore-court, gassed up, parked the car, and Sylvia and I went in search of some food. When we entered the restaurant, it became immediately evident that there were many intense discussions going on. As we were led to one of the few vacant tables, our waitress turned to us exclaiming, "It's awful, isn't it?"

"What is?" I asked.

"Haven't you heard about the wild dogs roaming around in huge packs and attacking people?" She pointed towards a window table. "The couple sitting over there saw them get two teenage boys riding their bikes near Gull Lake. They actually dragged the boys off the bikes and killed them. Other people have also seen some awful things. It's getting really scary."

I mentioned we had come in from Manitoba and had seen a few dogs, but nothing like the large packs she was describing."

"I'm not surprised," she replied. "These dogs seem to be coming into Saskatchewan from Alberta, where, apparently, they have been a real plague. I hear they are out of control, particularly in Central Alberta."

"That is real bad news," I told her, explaining that we were on our way to Calgary and would have to go through that area. She sympathised as she took our order.

We talked it over and decided that, come what may, we would just have to keep going. Our snack arrived and with it the additional piece of advice to be extra cautious going through the Maple Creek area. Apparently, that is where the largest packs had been sighted. Neither Sylvia nor I said much as we ate. It was enough that everyone else appeared to be chattering nervously. From the over-heard conversation, we were not the only ones to be headed west.

I paid the bill, and we returned to the car. Everyone we passed wished us good luck. It sounded as though we would need it.

Back on the highway, the very next area we would be passing through was Gull Lake, where the wild dogs had attacked the cyclists. Several times we thought we saw packs of them in the distance. Then suddenly, there they were! They were still some distance ahead, but they were definitely in our path. It was a huge pack, numbering perhaps forty or fifty dogs. The animals were just milling around on the highway. We covered the distance with our hearts in our mouth, but fortunately, right before we reached the pack, their attention was drawn away from the highway by two farm dogs, one a German shepherd and the other something like a Pit Bull.

We had to look the other way as we passed by. The farm dogs didn't stand a chance. The wild dogs only stood ten to twelve inches high, but they had a wide bulldog type stance and lethal looking teeth and jaws, which they did not hesitate to use.

Once we got beyond those repulsive, marauding animals, the prairie scene seemed almost pastoral, and we tried to forget what we had seen. The road ahead appeared to be clear, but for how long we could only guess. Mile after mile passed, and for the better part of half an hour, there was only the odd sighting of small groups of the off-white coloured dogs, and thankfully, none were on the road. I wondered how I would react if a pack did indeed block the highway and refuse to move. I would not turn around, so other than stopping and waiting them out, the only option would be to plough through them. That could get ugly, and I didn't want to think about it.

Gull Lake was now behind us, and we were fast approaching Maple Creek, the area we had been warned about. Everything seemed normal, however. The sky was blue and we could see clear to the horizon. It was a beautiful day and we were making good time. Surely nothing could go wrong. *I must have had a bad dream*, I thought. How else could I explain the nightmarish threat posed by the wild dogs?

Then I knew this was no dream. I saw something I will never forget. In the distance, the horizon was actually throbbing! Instinctively, I knew the movement was created by hordes of the off-white dogs. Sylvia had fallen into a comfortable sleep, no doubt lulled by the purring of the engine and the warmth of the day. That was good. *Maybe with luck we will get through the next part of the journey without her having to be alarmed*, I thought. Bracing myself, I drove on.

For the next fifty or so kilometres the road was clear. The marauding animals were very much in evidence, though, and it seemed only a matter of time before they would confront us. When we reached the western edge of Maple

Wild Dogs Attack

Creek, we encountered what we had dreaded. There were dogs all over the road—perhaps hundreds of them— and these were in no better humour than the ones we had seen earlier.

A pack of a dozen or more had encircled a couple walking their pet Scottie. We made it past, but what I saw in the rear-view mirror turned my stomach. More of the horrible off-white creatures had arrived on the scene, and as though pre-planned and co-ordinated, the whole mass launched a ferocious attack on the terrified puppy. Its owners were not spared either, and there was absolutely nothing anyone could do to help them.

I moved gingerly forward, and thankfully the dogs moved aside as I proceeded through the intersection. I saw their giving ground more as self preservation than backing down and was grateful for my large, solid car. On the other side of the intersection, a guy in a white convertible was fighting a losing battle against the dozens of dogs that were jumping into his car and viciously attacking him. Again, there was nothing I could do but keep going.

Slowly picking up speed, I continued working my way through the packs of animals. I took comfort in the fact that, by now, a number of other vehicles were also travelling west behind me. I was glad not to be alone and, fortunately, Sylvia had slept through the whole episode.

After leaving Maple Creek, there were fewer of the wild dogs, but we still had to be very vigilant. By the time we reached the Calgary city limits, I had struck and possibly killed three or four. In view of their sheer numbers, it was surprising I hadn't hit more of them.

51

I decided to stop in at the office, which was on the way home. By this time, we were again surrounded by numerous packs of the wild animals. They were on both sides of the highway, and when we turned off to approach the office parking lot, there were more of them on both sides of the road. In fact, there were dogs as far as the eye could see. The only exception was that there were no dogs in the parking lot itself, although there were a few across the road, and they seemed quite interested in our arrival.

Sylvia did not want to stay in the car by herself, so we decided we should both make a run across the ten or so yards between our car and the office door. I inched in a little closer, cutting the distance by about three yards. We agreed to exit the car on a count of three, then opened our doors simultaneously and made a dash for safety. We were just in time. As I got through behind Sylvia, the two lead dogs were throwing themselves against the now closing doors. That was too close for comfort.

Inside, there was pandemonium. Some of the wild dogs had broken in through a back door. They were, for the moment, contained, but we could hear them clawing and scratching and throwing themselves against walls and doors in search of a weak spot where they could break through.

Then we discovered they had a weak spot! On their forehead, centrally positioned above eye level, there was a protuberance. Several people had noted that if a dog was threatened with a stake or iron bar to the head, the animal would freeze, open it's eyes wide, and appear to say 'oh no, please don't'. One fellow was seen to take pity on a dog and back off. He did not have long to regret his decision. As soon as lowered his weapon, the animal leaped on him and sank its fangs into his throat.

If the dogs took a blow to the protuberance, however, they were instantly felled; so, everyone in the building had armed himself or herself with a stake or club of some sort.

Sylvia and I spent several hours helping the others beat off any dogs that broke through. After a while, things quieted down somewhat, and I decided we had better head for home. There was no telling what we would find there.

Choosing our moment carefully, Sylvia and I made a dash for our car and lost no time getting underway. It struck us as strange, but the farther south we travelled, the fewer wild dogs we encountered.

It took us about thirty minutes to get home. There were no wild dogs in sight. In fact, we had seen none for the last two or three kilometres. Very much relieved, Sylvia went indoors and I started to unpack the car. After what we had just experienced, the calm seemed very quiet and unreal. I had taken one load in and was in the midst of bringing in another when I heard a shout. I looked up just in time to see two of the ferocious dogs bearing down on me.

I darted towards the open front door and almost made it. Then, to my horror, I felt a searing pain in my right leg. That was the first indication that one of the dogs had drawn blood. I managed to reach the house and pulled the door closed behind me with not a second to spare. Safely inside, I limped into the kitchen to examine my injured leg. Sylvia took one look and insisted I got to the Emergency Room for treatment. After a brief moment's thought, I agreed and phoned for an ambulance.

Half an hour later, I was at Rockyview Hospital. I saw many of the nurses I knew from the Intensive Care Unit and figured they must have been called in because of the wild dog crisis. If I had imagined that, because I was an existing patient, they would come to my aid quickly, I was mistaken. Much to my annoyance, I had to wait my turn. I flagged down one of the nurses and tried to get some idea of how much longer I would have to be patient.

"Brian," she said sharply, "we have so many people here who are in much worse shape than you. We will be with you as soon as we can." I felt a little abashed at the upbraiding, but guess I deserved it.

I don't recall how long I had to wait, but finally, Stephanie came over and playfully scolded me for my impatience. She wheeled me over to another room where, with help, I was transferred to a bed. Once my wounds were cleaned and dressed, Stephanie called for a porter to take me back to Intensive Care. She must have wondered how I had managed to get my leg torn up by a wild dog without leaving the hospital, but she never asked.

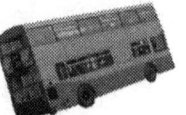

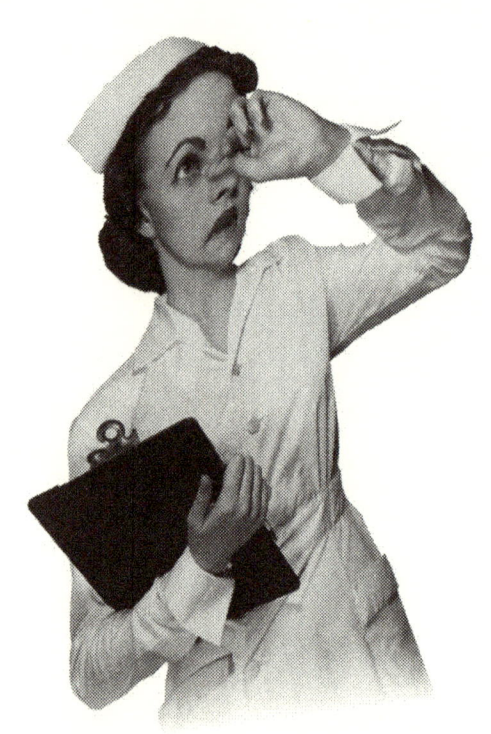

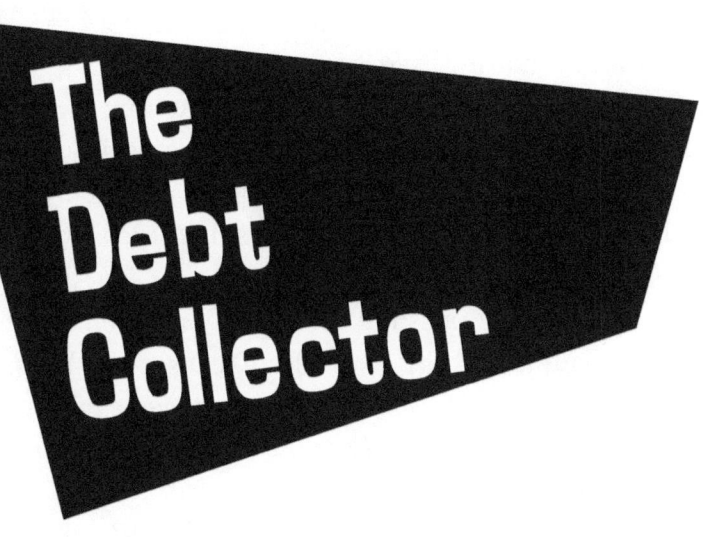

The Debt Collector

Someone had left a summary of the cost of my hospital stay on the notice board in my room. I could see it quite clearly from my bed and recall it being in the neighbourhood of $22,000—and that was just for the first month in the Rockyview Hospital!

Why had it been left there, I wondered? *Was it to remind me they needed my money?* Now I had something else to worry about. *Wasn't the province covering all health care costs? Did I have to come up with all this money? Surely not.*

For a time I was able to ignore the notice, feeling that if I did, the problem might go away. Several days passed and nobody referred to it. There were, of course, a number of other possibilities. Maybe the management simply wanted patients to know what the cost of their treatment and accommodation was; or maybe it was someone's idea of a joke.

My concern about the notice continued for the next few days. Then to make matters worse, a desk appeared just outside of my door, and eventually someone whom I did not recognise, sat there armed with papers and a variety of folders. She put a notice on her workstation that read, 'All accounts to be paid here'. *Now,* I asked myself, *why outside of my door? Has this been done for a reason?*

I imagined it would be possible for me to pay the costs for a month or so, but after that, it would take a serious bite out of our savings. *Perhaps if I could pay for just one month,* I reasoned, *I could stall them from throwing me out and manage to stay for one additional month.*

This problem had me worried for some time. Was it a dream, or reality?

Post Script: Dream or reality? It seems a little of both. Visitors to my ward later admitted to seeing a similar notice.

~ Author

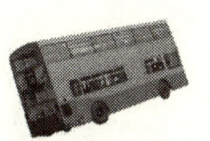

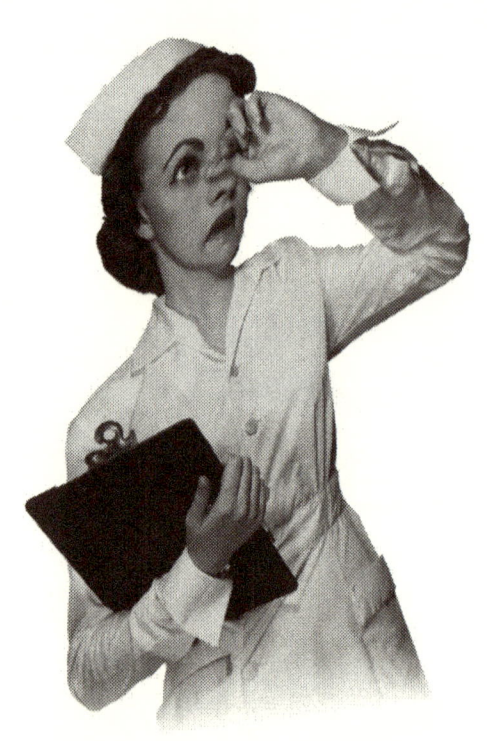

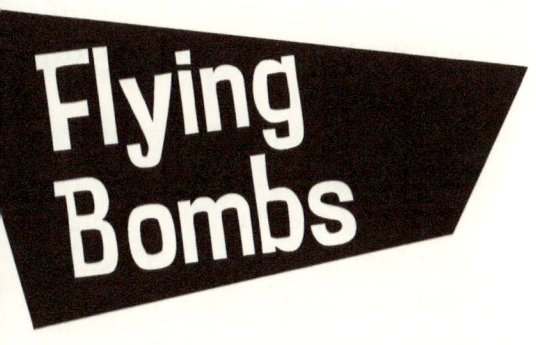

Flying Bombs

had successfully persuaded my wife to join me for a day's outing
to the mountains. The Rockies always provided a welcome
change from city living, and we had both been working
hard and were convinced we needed a short break. We
were approaching Banff on Highway 1. It was almost mid-
day, and we were starting to get hungry. Rounding a bend
in the road, we saw a most unusual sight. At the side of the
road was a huge billboard, unusual in that such advertising
was not normally permitted along the highway. It was pro-
moting a new low-cost aircraft, claiming that for fourteen
thousand dollars it was possible to acquire it. There was a
catch, though. Apparently, when the airplane ran out of
fuel—and for that price there was no fuel gauge — it would
go into a dive, and a nose first landing would be unavoid-

able. I was intrigued and stopped the car to take a closer look.

The product looked very much like a Second World War fighter jet and also something like a Mustang. I couldn't help being interested and made up my mind to visit the distributor's showroom when we returned from our trip.

By the time we arrived back in the city it was pretty late, but the showroom was still open so we stopped by and asked for a brochure. The salesman asserted we had little time to order since their product was in great demand. I assured him I bought absolutely nothing major without first sleeping on it, and this would definitely be considered a major purchase. He finally gave me a brochure, muttering about how few they had left.

Brochure in hand, we returned to the car and made our way home. The next morning, I took some time to examine the information on the new low-cost aircraft. It seemed to have exciting possibilities, in spite of its tendency to be a 'one-way ticket.' The small print indicated another problem. In addition to its proclivity for landing nose first, it seems the plane screeched like a dive-bomber. The noisemaking device couldn't be switched. To stop the racket, it had to be physically destroyed. To this end, the manufacturer had placed a small bomb in the nose of the aircraft, the cost of which was included in the selling price—thus the nickname, Flying Bombs.

The small print put me off, and I lost interest. Others, however, were obviously not deterred, for within a few weeks, the skies were full of screaming aircraft. It was hard

Flying Bombs

to ignore them. All you could do was wait and hope they didn't run out of fuel while overhead.

Some time later, we were shopping downtown and saw one of the Flying Bombs. According to other shoppers, it had been aloft for a while, and everyone was anxiously eyeing the sky. Suddenly we could hear the engine cut, and the plane went into a nosedive right above the shopping area. Either deliberately or as the result of a miscalculation, the pilot had obviously run out of gas. Who will ever know?

Thankfully, he missed hitting anything but hardtop, but I became absolutely convinced that I didn't want to buy one.

Post Script: No excuses offered for this one!

~ Author

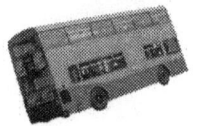

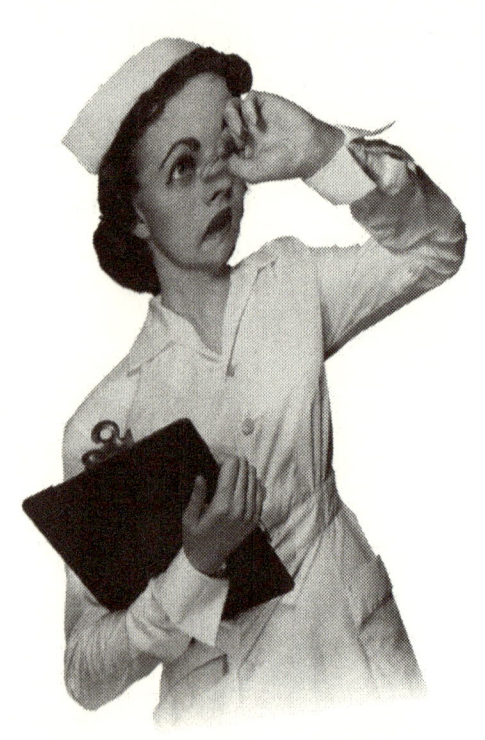

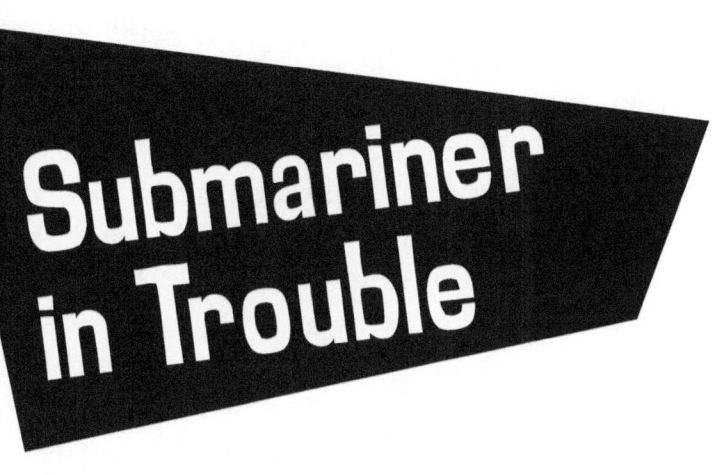

Submariner in Trouble

It was stuffy and dark. It was also late at night, and from the noises we must have been submerged, or so I thought. I was being accommodated in the hold of what appeared to be a large submarine. I didn't know how I got there or why, and it was impossible to ask, since I was totally unable to communicate. I was paralysed and totally reliant on the nurse in charge perceiving my needs. To expect answers to complicated questions such as "What am I doing here?" was not realistic.

I lay in my bunk, frustrated at my inability to move. A great deal of the time, I was uncomfortable. From time to time, instrument lights would flash, and occasionally, alarms would go off. Not that I minded the lights or the general confusion. Indeed, the more that was happening, the better my chances of being seen by a passing nurse.

My nurse, or at least the one I thought was mine, had a bunk in the same room. It had a drape, which could be pulled across for privacy. Whenever someone's alarm sounded, she would pull back her drape; get out of her bunk, and go check things out.

On this particular night, I had a brick, or something that felt like one, in my bed. I was lying on it! Now, if only an alarm would sound, maybe the nurse would come.

Paralysed or not, I could use my eyes, or so I thought, to signal my extreme discomfort. Still my chances of attracting attention were not good. I don't know how long I'd been there, but I couldn't remember the last time anyone had spoken to me, let alone come to adjust my bedding.

Suddenly another alarm sounded. It wasn't mine, but it was close enough that to investigate it, the nurse would have to walk right by my bunk. Finally, I might get lucky!

At first, there was movement in her bunk. Then, her drape moved to the side, and in the half-light, I saw her get out of bed, hurry along past my bunk without so much as a glance at me, and fumble around with one of the other patient's ventilators. Now if I were to attract her attention, it would have to be on her way back.

I was really getting desperate. If only I could cause something to fall to the floor that she would have to stop and pick up or that she would trip over. Of course, since I couldn't move, that was out of the question. I had to think quickly. What else could I do? Maybe I could move my head from side to side to let her know that there was a problem. Unfortunately, just because I felt that I could move my head didn't mean I actually was able to. I was aware that what I thought I was doing wasn't necessarily what was happening. Even so, I had to give it a try.

Sure enough, having solved the other patient's problem, the nurse returned to her bunk without even looking in my direction.

This would happen time and time again. I couldn't understand how the nurse could be unaware of my condition and my ongoing need of attention. Was she just choosing to do nothing? I can't remember how long I was ignored in this fashion or how I finally got out of the submarine. I did, however, have the thought that I was no good to the navy while incapacitated!

Post Script: This dream must have been experienced in Intensive Care, at the Foothills Hospital. I could not remember, but my wife later explained I was not in a single room, and that beds in that ward were separated by drapes, for privacy. No doubt the same drapes I observed in the submarine hold!

Even after nine or ten months of hospitalization, I could, on occasion, feel that my knees were bent and my lower legs were dangling through the bed, with my feet almost on the floor. It was impossible of course; I could still see my toes at the end of the bed! I never told anyone.

~ Author

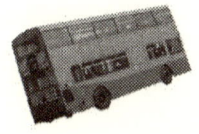

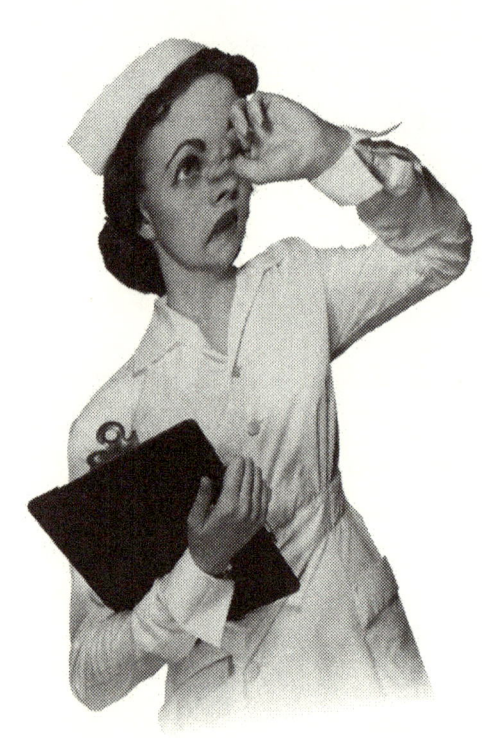

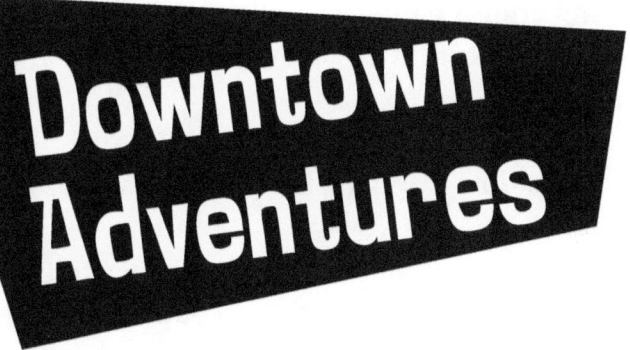

Downtown Adventures

Somehow I made it downtown again, and into the Plus Fifteen system, a system of above street level covered walkways and bridges connecting much of the downtown core.

It was getting rather late and was time to start looking for some accommodation. As it turned out, I didn't have very far to go.

I think it was somewhere near 9th Avenue that I saw a small hotel just off the Plus Fifteen. *That should be worth exploring,* I remember thinking. *I could be independent for once and avoid going back to the hospital.* I liked what I saw. It didn't look very expensive and appeared to offer suitable accommodations, so I booked in for later that evening and took some time to wander around.

The first stop was to be the bank, as I needed money. On the way, I heard what was becoming a very familiar sound. I was on one of the many bridges that criss-cross the downtown area. It had a stairwell that went to the roadway below, and I heard several cars using their new musical horns. It wasn't an unpleasant sound, although it could get annoying after a while. Actually, it made me feel as though I were on vacation in some other part of the world. Europe, perhaps.

Unfortunately, by the time I reached the bank it was closed. Now I had a problem.

With no cash, I was stuck. Sure I had a wallet full of plastic, but being unable to use my hands, I could not sign a receipt. I tried to think of a way around it. I had already booked my hotel room and given the clerk my credit card number, so perhaps I could arrange for my wife to meet me in the morning, and she could sign. It was worth a try.

I wandered around for a while longer and then decided to call it a night. I went back to the hotel, but to my surprise, things were a little different than they had been earlier in the day. For one thing, a whole area opposite the check-in counter had been opened up, revealing a number of single beds and a couple of washrooms with padlocks on the doors. Wait a minute, I thought. *I hope they are not going to give me one of those beds.*

Turning to the busy reception area, I signalled to one of the clerks and was politely asked to wait. I spent the next few minutes anxiously tapping out a rhythm on the counter. I feared the worst. There was a convention in the city, and it was soon obvious from the replies others were receiving that rooms were at a premium.

Downtown Adventures

When my turn came, I asked the clerk for my room key. He turned to the board, then, as though suddenly remembering something, he turned back to face me saying he was sorry, but I had been allocated one of the beds opposite the desk. "The rest of the hotel is fully booked," he explained, and seeing the look of amazement on my face, added, "There is not a room left anywhere in the city."

"But, there is no privacy in that area," I insisted.

"We have a screen that can be drawn across to separate that space from the reception area, and I will have that arranged immediately, sir."

I complained one more time, though I knew I would get nowhere.

"Sorry, sir. If we could do better, we would," was the only response I would get. He pointed to the bed allocated to me.

So it is either this or nothing, I thought.

"All right, I will take it," I said, Then I spun my chair around, wheeled into the area temporarily set aside for bedrooms, and dumped my belongings on the bed earmarked for me. I knew it would be too late to arrange for transportation to anywhere else. Somehow I made it under the covers and was able to fall asleep, but not before two thoughts crossed my mind. The first was *I wonder if the hospital staff will miss me tonight?* The second was *Why have they put padlocks on the washroom doors?*

I was soon to have the answer to that second question. I was awakened many times during the night by people coming and going, and much of the traffic seemed to consist of non-residents. Then there were the late night revellers using their musical car horns on the street below. A small window just above my bed opened up to what I guessed to be 10th Avenue. I finally decided further sleep was out of the question, so I had lots of time to worry about paying the hotel bill.

I planned to climb out of bed before anyone stirred. I would quietly get my belongings together and slip out of the main door without being seen. They would have my credit card number, so I hoped they would not accuse me of leaving without paying the bill. I would ask my wife to stop by later in the day and sign to settle the account.

It was a great plan in theory, but in spite of everything, I must have fallen asleep again. When I woke up, there was a bustle of activity and the sun was high in the sky. I clearly had to change my plan. I would have to talk my way out of this situation. Then something quite unexpected happened. Someone was tugging at my arm.

"I am having difficulty locating your vein," I heard the white-coated woman say. "I am going to leave this to the doctor."

On looking around it was soon obvious that I was in my bed in Intensive Care. So I had not managed to avoid going back to the hospital, after all.

The next night was different. This time I really was going downtown. I made it in my traveling bedstead to the mezzanine in one of the centrally located office towers. Luckily, I had help getting on and off a public elevator, into which my bed fit with only an inch to spare; otherwise I wouldn't have made it to the second floor. The occasion was an exhibition, which I did not want to miss. I ran into a number of people I knew and could spend time talking to.

The evening passed quickly, and it was soon time to leave. I was just about to call it a day, when I spotted one of my nurses, Betsy. She looked most surprised to see me there.

"Brian, you should not be out of the hospital!" she exclaimed.

"Why not?" I asked. "Nothing is happening there, and I am never missed. And there is so much to do here." Then as an afterthought: "Are you going back there now?"

"No," she said. I am one of the organizers and expect to be here until well after midnight."

We talked for quite a while. Finally she excused herself to get some work done, and I decided to leave. A janitor came to my rescue and pushed my bed towards the elevators. As we got closer, he paused, and reminded me that the public elevators were closed for the night. Scratching his head, he wondered out loud how I could exit the building. He eventually decided he would have to leave me where I was and seek help.

I waited for quite a while. In the end, Betsy came across me again and, upon realizing my predicament, offered to help. She remembered there was a service elevator in the back and thought we could use that. *Thank goodness*, I thought. It would not be much fun to be trapped in here for the night.

With the help of the janitor, we made it to the ground floor and then outside. It was cold, and I shivered as I thanked my rescuers. I hoped one of the familiar white R.T.[1] trucks would soon arrive to give me a lift.

It was starting to snow very lightly, but enough so that after a few minutes my bed was covered. Fortunately, it was the dry stuff, otherwise my sheets would have been soaking wet. Thankfully, I did not have long to wait. The R. T. truck driver must have spotted me from over half a block away, as he very smoothly changed lanes and pulled up just ahead of me. "Look," he said, "I can't take you straight back because I'm on my way to a party. Would you like to come with me? You will know most of the guys there. My name is Malcolm, by the way."

Without a moment's hesitation I agreed, which I think is what he expected; and he loaded me on as though this were purely routine.

We drove for about fifteen minutes, then turned into the driveway of a large mansion. "What are you doing here?" I questioned. "This is the home of the city police chief, and it is not likely he would be holding a party for us."

"Don't worry," Malcolm replied. "I believe he is out of town. It's his daughter who is throwing the party. She is one of the nurses from the hospital. You probably know her."

The front door was unlocked, so in we went. Moving through the crowd of people who were already there, we made our way to the kitchen, figuring out where it was by observing where the food was coming from. Then from somewhere behind me, I heard a familiar voice, "Hi Brian, glad you made it." I spun around to see a nurse named Clara.

---

1 In my dreams, I imagined respiratory therapists — R.T.'s — all had large white trucks containing a laboratory and all of their equipment, for mobility. In reality, no such trucks existed!

"I need to sit down," I told her. She looked around and quickly came to the conclusion the safest thing would be to take me up the stairs at one side of the kitchen, which seemed to lead nowhere except to a series of upper storage cupboards. At the top was a seat, which could be unfolded from the wall.

She has to be joking, I thought hopefully. But, this was no joke. Clara, it seemed, was not above giving me a bad time. She had arranged for volunteers to assist me up the stairs, giving me little option but to do her bidding. Everyone else in the kitchen, and Clara's boyfriend in particular, area seemed highly amused at my predicament. There I was, stuck up in the air, feeling like a fool. Upon closer investigation, I realized the boyfriend looked familiar. Then it hit me that virtually every guest was an employee of our largest competitor, and they were really enjoying seeing their competition having a bad time.

Everyone except me was enjoying the party. I watched as supper was prepared in the kitchen below me. Clara was close by loading a tray of fresh fruit. I called to her over the din and asked if her father was aware of this party in his absence. She gave me a look that told me it was not a good question to ask.

What had happened, I wondered, *to make Clara so antagonistic towards me?* She was always so friendly and helpful at the hospital, but not so now. *Maybe it was boyfriend trouble or maybe her father was coming home unexpectedly.* I had no chance to converse with her, so there wasn't much hope of getting answers.

I was getting tired of being the butt of jokes in the kitchen. Also, by this time, I was really sleepy.

Finally, Malcolm, whom I had not seen since our arrival, came to the rescue. "Let's go and find you a chesterfield," he said. "There's no way we will be leaving here tonight." I was only too happy to agree.

Within half an hour, I was in a spacious lounge. I'd been bathed and placed on the owner's favourite and expensively covered chesterfield. It wasn't the best place for a patient in my condition, but I was too tired to argue.

I awoke with a start. It must have been the following afternoon. I was still on the same chesterfield, but now I was surrounded by what appeared to be family members and friends of Clara. Some were quietly talking, others were reading, and a few were knitting. Clara noticed I was awake and, with none of the previous night's antagonism, asked if I were okay. *Was the party last night just a dream?* I wondered.

Without waiting for my reply, she added, "Malcolm just phoned, and he will be here to pick you up in about an hour. It's snowing pretty hard — almost a white out — and there have been a lot of accidents. It's a pity you have to go out in this weather."

I wondered how they were going to transfer me into the truck, but I was grateful to be someplace warm and dozed off again.

Next thing I knew someone was gently shaking my arm and saying, "Wake up, wake up! It's time to get you in your chair." It was one of my nurses, and I was in my room in Intensive Care. *How did Malcolm get me back without waking me?*

Downtown Adventures

"Did you just change the sheet?" I asked. "The other one must have been wet from the snow."

The nurse gave me a funny look. She must have thought I'd been dreaming!

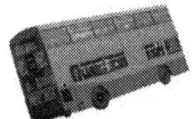

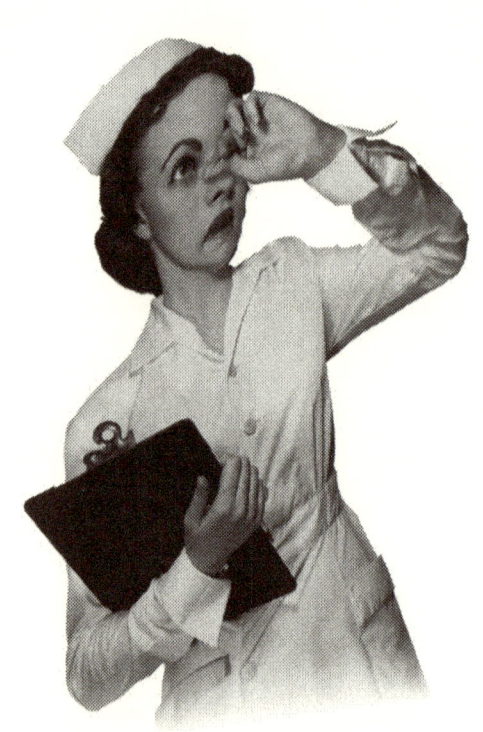

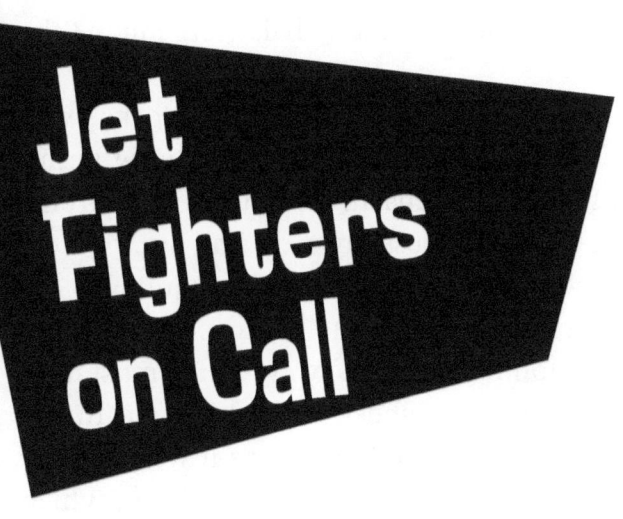

Jet Fighters on Call

It was a beautiful warm day in early fall. There were eight or nine jet fighters parked, nose first, in the trees opposite my hospital room. Backed by tall conifers, some of the trees had been planted when the grounds of the hospital were initially landscaped a good number of years ago. Mostly they were green-leafed varieties, including some heavily berried Mountain Ash; but there were also quite a number of a red-leafed variety, and it was these that the jet pilots seemed to prefer to use as their stand-by locations.

The pilots, in goggles and full flying gear, were either sitting in their aircraft or standing on a branch alongside. In any event, they were ready for action. How they backed out and made their way to a runway when the call came, I never knew. I did see how they landed, though. They'd come straight into a tree and stop, perfectly balanced, among the branches!

I had heard there was a new airport a few blocks away and wondered if this were some kind of publicity stunt. Since Sylvia and I would be departing from the new airport on a trip to Spain, we would possibly soon find out.

Time passed, and it was another sunny day, quite hot for the time of year. We made our way to the airport. We were walking, and it was uphill most of the way, which must have been tough for Sylvia, since she was pushing me in my wheelchair. We hadn't booked a flight, since it was cheaper to take advantage of the airline's introductory plan, which involved simply entering your names at check-in for the next flight to your destination. There was a snag, though.

This introductory offer applied only to six-seater twin-engine aircraft; so, allowing for a pilot, that left room for five passengers. If more than five people were listed for a flight, a drawing would be held to determine who could board.

When Sylvia and I arrived at the check-in desk, we were directed to wait in the lounge. Imagine our surprise when we spotted two of our friends there, also waiting for a flight to Spain. We enjoyed the great view and basked in the sunshine that was streaming in through the large windows. I was so comfortable that I fell asleep.

The next thing I remember was being gently awakened. The sun was still shining, but something was different. When I looked out the window, the trees with the red leaves and the Mountain Ash loaded with their red berries were still there, but no airport. The jet fighters that had been parked in the trees had also disappeared, and I was no longer in a wheelchair, but back in the hospital again. I don't know what happened to our trip to Spain!

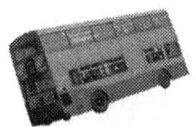

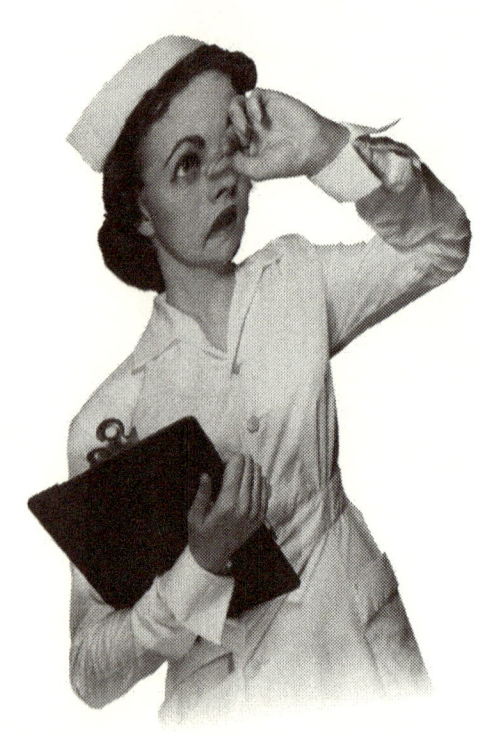

Catastrophe

It was one of those ordinary Sundays. Sylvia and I had decided to take a short drive and find somewhere different to enjoy a leisurely cup of coffee. The weather, though, was anything but ordinary. The day had started sunny and warm, but then turned thundery. Next a weather system came through, bringing high winds followed by lots of rain. Before long, the temperature dropped, and the rain changed to sleet. Finally, it started to snow.

As we set off, the sun was peeking through the clouds, but with all the moisture in the air, it was becoming quite misty. In fact, before we had travelled very far, the weather forecasters would probably be calling it 'fog.' We decided not to venture too far, and headed for the Midnapore Railway Station, where there was a reasonably good restaurant on the upper level.

Arriving at the station, which actually no longer served as one since passenger trains didn't come through anymore, I parked the car. By this time visibility was perhaps only a hundred yards or so. We made our way inside, hoping that by the time we came out, things would have improved.

In the station, very little was left on the ground floor except an empty ticket office and waiting room. We were just about to head up the flight of concrete steps that led to the second floor restaurant, when I had a strange sense of foreboding. Maybe this was not a good idea. I was about to suggest we choose another restaurant when my attention was drawn to a lady who appeared somewhat distressed. Sylvia noticed her too. We went to offer assistance.

"How can we help?" Sylvia asked as we approached her.

"My car has broken down," she told us in broken English. "I am a visitor to this country and thought I would be able to continue my journey by train."

"No passenger trains travel this line," I explained. "This building hasn't functioned as a station in years. It serves a different purpose now."

"No one told me that," she sighed. "I have been waiting since early this morning."

This made our next decision easy. "Please allow us to buy you some food and a warm drink," I offered. Afterwards I will drive you to the Greyhound Bus Terminal."

The lady gratefully accepted the offer and asked us to wait while she went back to her car for something. No sooner had she left us than we heard the unmistakable sound of powerful diesel engines rumbling towards us

84

through the fog. Soon we could make out a headlight, and the ground was starting to vibrate. I could not help but be in awe of the huge locomotives that were capable of hauling so much freight, particularly when lashed together in threes and fours, as trains on this line so often were.

I hoped the lady, whose name we still had not discovered, would have the good sense to stay on her side of the track until the train passed by. It couldn't be far away now, but the fog made it difficult to judge just how close it was. Soon the noise was pounding at the eardrums, and the ground was trembling under the weight and momentum of the heavy diesels. The train was now emerging from the fog and approaching the station fairly rapidly, no doubt picking up speed as it was leaving the city.

Both Sylvia and I stood watching as the first of the locomotives thundered through. It was an impressive sight. Then came the repetitive sounds of the freight cars passing by. I had, on many previous occasions, counted one hundred or more in a single train, and this one seemed to be no exception. We decided to head up the stairs to the restaurant, thinking we would find a table, then, after the freight had passed, I could come down to find the lady we had offered to help.

On entering the restaurant, there was a tremendous noise, and the whole building shook violently. I ran down the stairs to see what was happening and, to my amazement, saw that one of the freight cars had a wide load that had not only hit the side of the building, but had lifted it off its foundation and was dragging it along, carrying us down the track like a projectile. I considered making a jump to safety, but couldn't do that without Sylvia, so I let the opportunity pass. We were now traveling at a high speed, as if caught in a huge spinning top, yet the inside where we were, was absolutely stationary.

I rushed back upstairs, where there was something of a pandemonium. Everyone was looking out the windows in utter disbelief. Here we were in an urban restaurant, yet the rest of the world was rushing by at an alarming speed. The rail line from Midnapore going south was on a downhill gradient. The engineer, who I doubted had any knowledge of the extra baggage he'd picked up, was increasing power, and we were now travelling like a bullet.

For about twenty kilometres we moved in a line that was more or less straight. Then the track curved westward. It was at this point that the train and the station parted company. When the locomotive banked into the curve, the station continued in the direction it had been going, and was now sailing along on its own without any loss of speed.

We had no idea where this was all going to end. Prospects became darker when the restaurant manager turned on the radio just in time to hear a news bulletin on the 'Midnapore Disaster'.

"Hope is not yet lost for those trapped inside the station," the voice on the radio announced, "though the building is now traveling south-south east, leaving a trail of destruction in its wake. Officials say chances of a successful rescue operation are becoming increasingly remote, but experts are doing their best to come up with a plan."

That was how the general populace was learning of our

predicament. They were told the likelihood was that we would finish up in a small lake or river and be unable to exit the building. The anchorman explained that the best-case scenario was that the building would end up in the marshes where the water wasn't deep enough to cause drowning, but that the occupants might starve before rescuers could reach them. Although the outlook seemed pretty grim, we were trying to remain upbeat.

There were ten other people, including the restaurant's day manager, on board this fast moving projectile. Interestingly, almost everyone had a story about how they almost didn't choose this restaurant on this particular day. Only one elderly couple appeared resigned to their fate. To relieve the tension, the manager announced that all food and drink were now on the house. It did help a little. Then someone spotted a rescue helicopter flying overhead. That was good to see, although we realized not much could be done until we came to rest somewhere.

On and on we went, though we were losing some speed. I looked out the window in time to see us smash through the gate at a railway crossing and then careen down a well-traveled roadway. Thankfully we avoided hitting any cars. I decided to check out the damage downstairs, and scope things out just in case we needed a quick exit once this thing stopped. The manager agreed we should be prepared and offered to come with me.

We went through the swinging doors and cautiously made our way down the first flight of stairs. Everything looked normal until we got to the landing midway down. There we confronted by chaos. Where the outer doors used to be there was nothing but soil, vegetation, tree branches, rocks, and other debris that had been collected on our devastating run. There was no sign of the doors themselves, nor could we see any possible escape route. The exit was totally plugged.

"I've seen enough," I told the manager. "Let's see how we end up when we stop. If we come to a violent halt, perhaps enough damage will be done to give us an escape route."

He agreed, obviously hoping, as I was, that escape would be possible in the end. "What shall we tell the others?" he asked me.

"Lets tell them the truth — that it's a mess down here and we won't know much until we see how we finish up. Who knows? In the end, there may be several escape routes open to us."

The bizarre trip seemed endless. Now we were obviously on the prairie, since everywhere we looked, the land was flat and featureless. Our speed was still decreasing, but slowly; and the end of our run was nowhere in sight. We had no idea what was powering our movement now that we were free of the freight train.

The radio program was again interrupted to update listeners on our plight. It was eerie to be hearing the details of a catastrophe of which we were a part. Our path was apparently being tracked via reports phoned in by the ranchers and farmers whose properties we were crossing. Speculation was rife that the station would end up in the Drumhead Marshes, which would make rescue extremely difficult, if not impossible. We tried not to dwell on such a gloomy thought. "Anything could happen," we told ourselves.

Suddenly the scenery changed. We appeared to be headed into a large gully, and the level tabletop of the prairie was now above us. The deeper we went, the wider apart were the defining walls. It was beginning to appear that the gully was turning into a much larger canyon. The references on the radio to our finishing up in the marshes or in a lake now seemed to make sense.

As we headed downward into the canyon we must have gained some momentum, but we were now starting to level out again. Hopefully that meant we would be slowing down. I noticed the ground cover was becoming lush, which indicated the presence of moisture. I wondered if this were the marshy country that had been referred to in the radio alerts. It seemed we were about to find out.

The ride was becoming decidedly smoother at this point. Then, without any warning, everyone was thrown violently across the restaurant. Finally, we had stopped. A quick check turned up no major injuries, though most of us were hurting.

Now we had to find an escape route. I went to the doors and found them jammed, but when several of us charged with our shoulders, one of them swung aside. I ran through and headed down the stairs. As I had hoped, we'd gone into a rocky outcrop and the force of the collision had split one of the outside walls. There appeared to be enough space to crawl through. *But what about the ground outside,* I wondered? I decided to check it out, which proved to be a good decision. After making my way to the gap and peering out, all I could see was water. It was difficult to judge how deep it was and that presented a definite problem, but I calculated that we could not be far from the rocks and dry land.

I turned to the manager, who had come to look for himself.

"There must be a broom in the cleaning cupboard," I suggested. "We could use it to check the depth of the water." He agreed and offered to get it.

We soon determined that the water was about three feet deep. Now it might be possible to make plans. By this time, everyone had come to view the potential escape route, but it was soon agreed we should wait and see if rescuers came. Our wild ride had obviously been monitored so our whereabouts would soon be known, if we hadn't already been spotted.

Then someone shouted, "Look! Water is coming in."

Sure enough, water was now pouring in through the split in the wall. This was a new and worrisome development. Everyone must have been thinking, as I was: *How deep are we going to settle? Could it block our escape route?* It was then that one of the girls on the restaurant level spotted our would-be rescuers through the window.

We would still have to wait a while, but a party of six or seven was, indeed, scaling down an escarpment towards us. They were carrying planks and an assortment of ropes so their progress was rather slow. In the meantime, I tried to get a fix on where we were from the radio, but unfortunately, when we crashed it had fallen to the floor and no longer worked.

Catastrophe

It took some time for us all to evacuate the station, but eventually, with the assistance of our rescuers and their equipment, we waded through three feet of water to relatively dry land. We made our way along the base of the cliff, which led us to a fault in the side of the canyon, and from there, through a cutting where we were able to climb to the upper level.

Upon reaching the prairie, we saw that situated in a depression about half a mile away was a hotel that had an excellent view of the canyon. That was a pleasant surprise, or so it appeared at the time. *We can surely get help there,* I thought. I mentioned it to our rescuers and they agreed. We needed dry clothes and, more importantly, needed to shower. Wading waist deep in muddy water had left its mark on all of us. *Surely in view of our predicament, the hotel management would not refuse to help.*

The closer we got, however, the more obvious it became that we were looking at a luxury resort. That raised the question as to whether an upscale establishment would want to accommodate such a rag tag group as we. We would soon find out. There was very little alternative, so we had to press on and take our chances. By this time our clothes had thoroughly dried, but the evidence of our wading through the marsh could not be so easily hidden.

We reached the hotel entrance and decided to bite the bullet and enter the lobby. I saw the look on the face of one of the receptionists as we approached. It was not encouraging. She immediately came out from behind the front desk and hustled us into a side office. When we explained what had happened she looked like she didn't believe us. "We are fully booked for the season," she said with a somewhat icy tone. "The only rooms in which we could accommodate you are the staff quarters in the basement."

It was getting late, and we were all tired. "That's good enough for me," I responded. "As long as there is a bed to sleep on, I will gladly take one of the staff rooms." Everyone else echoed my sentiments, and after the receptionist cleared the arrangements with her manager, we were led downstairs to our respective rooms.

It did not take long to fall asleep that night.

Suddenly, I could feel someone gently shaking my shoulder. I opened my eyes, looked up, and saw a nurse. "Wake up, it's time for your blanket bath." Just for a moment, I wondered where I was. Then I realized I was back in my hospital room. I did not remember who had brought me back or how. Another thing puzzled me. How was it that no one appeared to miss me or, if they did, once again chose to say nothing about it? Don't they check the beds for patients every night?

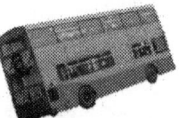

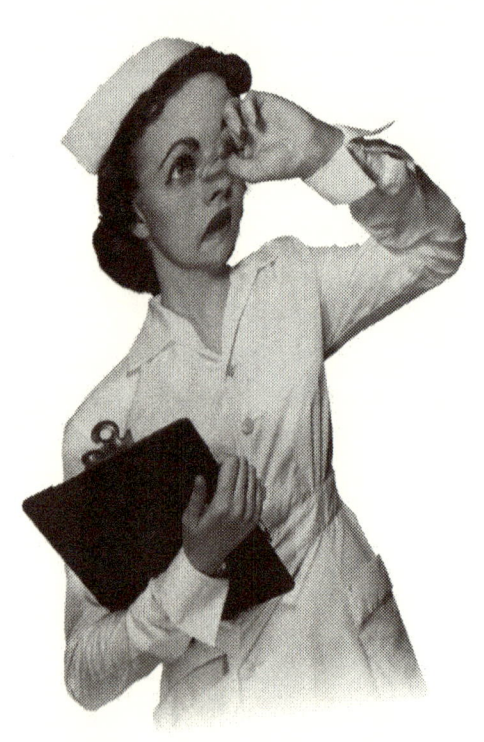

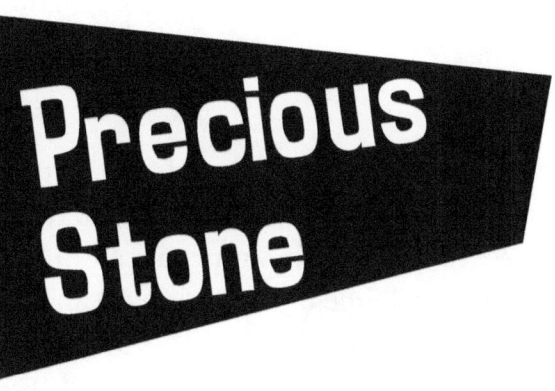

Precious Stone

Now, on top of everything else, I had cancer, or so I was told. I surmised, however, that I did not have to worry, because the malignancy I had was in the form of a very rare stone or crystal. I think it was in my bladder, but no one seemed too sure. This particular specimen, though, was very rare, and scientists needed a sample to keep for posterity.

Without wasting much time, I was duly prepared to travel to an army hospital in the bush. Some of the world's best scientists were either based there or associated in some way with the military establishment. My preparations included getting a shave, having my sheets changed, and having my hospital bed wheeled out and parked in the corridor. That was it. After half an hour or so, porters came and proceeded to wheel me out of the hospital. We continued across the grounds, and proceeded to the point where the main road entered the jungle. Then they just left me.

After another long wait, a great cloud of dust rose up from the dirt road. A military convoy was approaching, and it halted alongside me. I was rather unceremoniously loaded, and off we went.

Some time later, I awoke to see a white-coated doctor and a nurse holding up a jar containing their prize. It appeared to be quite a gemstone. "We discovered this rare cancer stone in your bladder," the doctor exclaimed. "Thought you might like to see it! Quite something isn't it?"

"Anyway," he went on, "We have you all stitched up again, and you're quite clear. We'll have you back to Intensive Care in your own hospital tomorrow after you've had a good sleep."

I should have billed them for the gemstone, I thought. Then: *What happened to the promise to get me back?* I was again on the dirt road where I had been picked up by the convoy. Although it was not getting dark yet, large crowds were congregating. My wife appeared through the crowd and joined me.

What is going on? I asked her. There were so many people around, and the crowd kept growing.

"Look at the images that are appearing," she answered, pointing to the western sky. "It's like a huge canvas of a moving pictures."

I was in awe at the wonderful sight. Imagine being in an open-air theatre with the sky as the stage and the clouds performing an absolute spectacle. It was sublime. Then, suddenly the weather changed. First the wind kicked up, eradicating the calm, and before long, the beautiful sky scenes were disappearing behind huge clouds of dust. The wind kept increasing in strength until the air was so dense with fine sandy particles that it was impossible to see. Everything that wasn't anchored down was being tossed around like so many pieces of paper. I covered my head with the bedclothes to keep from choking.

When the wind subsided a little, I peered out and saw that order was gradually appearing out of the chaos. But where was Sylvia? I looked around, but she was nowhere to be seen. Behind me was a large tented area, which I was sure hadn't been there before the storm. Or had it? *It could have been,* I reasoned, for we were, after all, quite close to the city.

Through one of the openings, I could look into the tent and see an enquiry desk, which I thought might be a good place to start looking for my wife. A kindly looking young fellow was passing, and I called to him and asked if he would mind pulling me over to the tent. He readily agreed, and once there, I was politely told by one of the staffers that I had to wait my turn. After some time, a matronly woman came over to me and asked how she could help. I asked if anyone had been looking for me, or if anyone had seen my wife. Apparently they had not. I was beginning to get a little alarmed. Not only had no one had seen Sylvia, but there was no transportation in sight to get me back to the hospital.

Another staff member came along and suggested I was in the way and should be moved. Without waiting for a response, he pushed me into a dingy looking building on the other side of the tented area. "We will let you know when anyone enquires for you," he promised as he left me to my own devices. I found myself in a small room, furnished with only a single bed and a cane table. It was hardly the Ritz. *Let me get out of here,* I thought. *But to where? I have no way of getting to the hospital or to a decent hotel.* I didn't have any money; I had just had an operation; and I was tired. With these thoughts going through my head, I fell asleep.

It must have been several hours later when I felt someone pulling at my shoulder. It was totally dark outside. "You mustn't miss the bazaar. I'll have you transferred to a chair and wheel you around. You have to spend something or you cannot stay." These words were muttered into my ear before I had even turned around to see who was there.

"Look," I tried to say; but I couldn't speak. *How can I let this guy know I have just had an operation?* I wondered. I couldn't even turn over to see who was addressing me.

At that moment I heard Sylvia's voice. She had Ruth with her, and they had obviously tracked me down, thankfully, just in time to help. They explained my predicament to the guy, who then pressed a small package into my hands. For some reason, I presumed it contained various good luck charms. There was a snag, though. Once the charms were accepted, the recipient was required to do favours for a group of what I believed to be religious fanatics. What those favours might be was anyone's guess, but they could be requested at any time. The sinister aspect was, the man explained, that ill fortune would befall me if I refused the charms.

Ruth suggested I raise my eyebrows once if I wished to accept the gift. I didn't hesitate. I raised my eyebrows twice.

Neither Ruth nor Sylvia approved of my choice. They were concerned about the possible implications. I was not about to be intimidated, though, and kept my hand open for the guy to take his lucky charms back. To my utter amazement, he reached for the small plastic container, tore it open, threw the contents on my bed, and stormed out.

I was destined to find small, cheap, prickly little souvenirs of that event in my bed for weeks to come. There were no precious stones, though.

My visitors, who had timed their arrival perfectly, were now offering to wheel my bed back to the hospital. I considered myself lucky. This was one of the few times I was actually looking forward to going back.

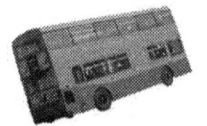

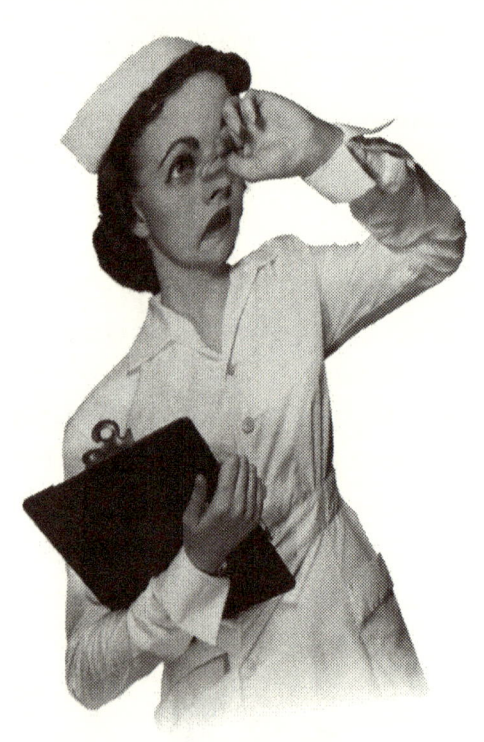

Quicksand Floor

My bed was going to be moved with me in it. That was a little scary. Whenever it was my turn to be moved, it was usual for me to be left — read that abandoned — in the 'halfway ward' with the unstable floor. I think there was only one such ward, and it overlooked the reservoir. From its window, you could see Woodson's Department Store, which was next to the hospital.

Sure enough, that is exactly where I was left. The nurse uttered the official mantra, "I will be back in two minutes," and continued on her merry way. Two minutes passed, then three, four, five minutes, and I was still alone. Fifteen minutes passed and still no sign of the nurse. Everything was all right for a while, but then I noticed the top of the bed appeared to be sinking. My head was lower than my feet. I peered over the edge of the bed and, to my dismay, saw that the upper end of it was most definitely sinking. Although, for the moment, the bottom still seemed on firm ground, I was terrified of being slowly swallowed up by the heaving, bubbling floor. It was as if my bed were standing in quick sand.

Where was everyone? No one had passed by since I'd been there, and there was no sign of my nurse. This was starting to feel serious. Then, just as the bed had sunk to a dangerous list, along came a nurse, who saw my predicament and rushed over. Two people, one a male nurse, responded to her pleas for help. They struggled mightily to lift the bed legs out of the floor, but with no result. The load had to be lightened; so together they lifted me off the bed and deposited me in a wheelchair in the corner.

To me, this was tremendously upsetting, although the nurses seemed to be taking it in stride. They retrieved the bed and moved it clear of the sinking floor. The male nurse asked me if I were all right and, without waiting for an answer, told me he would put a call out for my nurse, who should be back soon. With that, all three left the room, leaving me in the wheelchair.

It wasn't more than a couple of minutes before the floor around me again started to churn and heave. The spot under the right wheel of my wheelchair started to give way under my weight, and it wasn't long before the chair, with me in it, developed an ominous tilt. Since I couldn't use my arms, moving away was not an option. I was terrified.

"Nu-u-u-u-rse," I called as loudly as I could, "nu-u-u-u-rse, please!" Nothing happened. There was no response. Meanwhile, I was sinking deeper. The right wheel of my chair was already buried up to the axle, and the other one was now sinking, as well. I felt justified in panicking! I called out again, even louder than before.

Just when I had given up hope of anyone responding, in walked my regular nurse. She took one look at me huddled in my half-buried wheelchair and stepped back in horror. Then she pulled herself together and called for help. Another nurse came in immediately, and together they tugged at my chair until finally the wheels broke free of the floor's grip.

Another four nurses were rounded up, and the six of them transferred me back into the bed.

"Don't leave me here," I pleaded. "Park me anywhere else, but don't leave me here!" I breathed a sigh of relief as my original nurse took hold of the foot of the bed and we were on our way. We no sooner reached the doorway, however, when a 'code blue' was announced over the intercom. My nurse quickly pushed me into another room, where I found myself amongst wing chairs, sofas, and love seats. This room was obviously part of Woodson's Furniture Store. Not again, I thought, as once again I found myself alone.

The trouble with the code system is that the patient being left for another whose needs are desperately urgent, never knows how long he will have to wait before someone comes back for him.

Although I saw nary a nurse, I could hear members of Woodson's staff passing by the storeroom where I'd been left. As time passed, my fear of being alone returned. It was a concern that was never very far away, but on this occasion, it was acute. It got more so, as I suddenly realized how very quiet it had gotten. Now, I felt sure I had been forgotten. Although I couldn't know for certain, I thought the code blue must have either been cancelled or completed. It had been a long time, and still no one had come. Finally I heard a key turn. My heart soared, and then sank just as fast. The door to my room was not being opened. It was being locked! I just knew I had been forgotten.

I had to do something. Though I felt a little groggy, I struggled out of the bed and made my way to the only window. With great difficulty, I managed to slide it open just enough to squeeze through. I dropped to the ground and found myself in the hospital's parking lot. I proceeded painfully towards a white Mobile Emergency Respiratory Assistance truck. Blessedly, it wasn't locked, and I climbed into the cab to find the keys had carelessly been left in the ignition. I gave just a moment's thought to driving away, to going home for the first time in ages, but decided I should wait for the driver and try to persuade him to take me. I desperately hoped it would be one of the guys that I knew.

Not knowing how long I would have to wait, I lay across the seat and tried to relax. The driver was not long coming. Not only wasn't he a friend of mine, but when he saw me, he became pretty belligerent.

"Caught you!" he exclaimed as if I were a vagrant. "You were just about to steal my truck, right?"

I tried to collect my composure. I was sure this driver must have been employed by 'the competition' (one of the other hospitals). I knew I was in deep trouble when my protest fell on deaf ears. His mind was obviously made up, and nothing I could say was going to change that. "I could call the police," he said, "but that would take time I don't have. I have a busy night, so I am taking you home with me until I decide what to do with you." I was in no condition to argue and imagined I would be better off to quietly comply, at least for the time being.

About twenty minutes later, we pulled into his driveway. Two children ran out to meet him followed by a woman I presumed was his wife. After shooting me an angry look, he swung out of the truck, slamming the door behind him. He then got into a heated conversation with the lady, pointing occasionally in my direction. When Don, as I heard her call him, returned to the truck, he told me, "We are transferring you to the chesterfield in our family room. You will have to stay there until I get home later tonight. Then we will figure out what we are going to do with you."

At least, I now had the prospect of being reasonably comfortable for the next few hours. The children were eyeing me with curiosity as they ran in and out of the room in play. Time passed. There were few other distractions. There was a television, but it was hidden from my view by a room divider. After what seemed like two hours or so, Don's wife came in. To my utter amazement, she started to sprinkle two-inch nails onto the unoccupied part of the chesterfield. I took this as a hostile act. I no longer had any illusions. I was in enemy territory.

For the rest of the evening, I was left pretty well to myself. I certainly felt threatened, but more than that, I was frustrated. Physically unable to get up and out of there, I had no alternative but to await the return of the 'master'. It was, perhaps, the longest evening I have ever spent.

Finally, around eleven Don returned. I could hear voices coming from the direction of the kitchen; then both he and his wife appeared at the doorway. "We are on duty tonight. We both have to go, so we are going to take you and drop you off at your place," Don asserted. With that, they helped me up from the chesterfield and carried me, somewhat clumsily, to the truck, where, after much pushing and shoving, they place me on the bunk over the driver's cab. I lay there while they packed their belongings, got on board, and drove away.

I found the truck's movement very calming — so much so, I must have been asleep within minutes. How long I slept, I don't know, but when I awoke I was in the familiar surroundings of Intensive Care, and a nurse's aide was offering me a warm blanket. I remembered nothing of how I got back there, and everyone acted as though I had never left the place; so I said nothing.

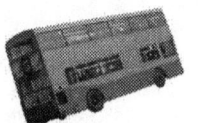

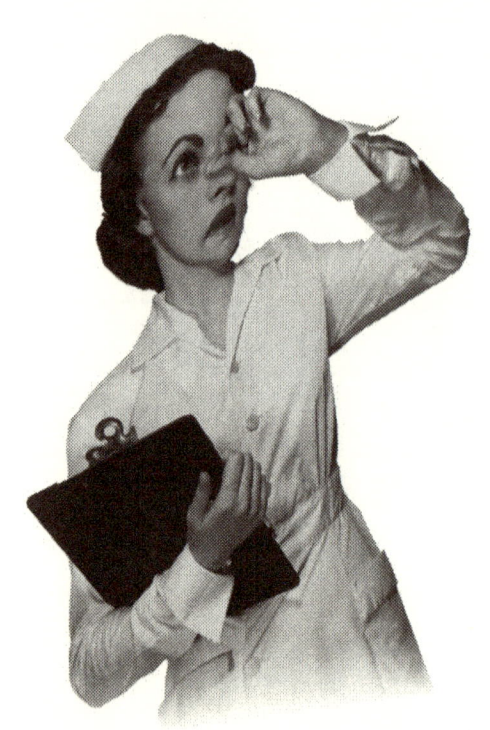

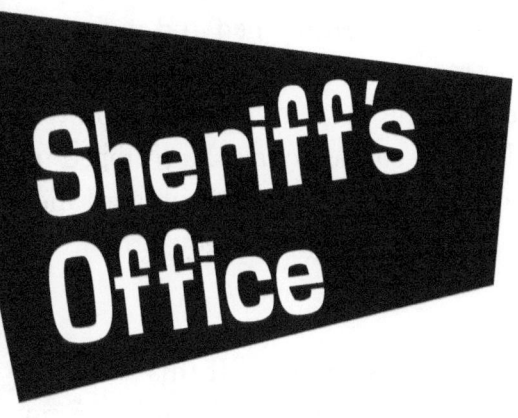

Sheriff's Office

The sun must have been pretty low in the afternoon sky because the shadow on the floor-to-ceiling window was quite clear. From my bed I could see the outline of someone wearing a cowboy hat and boots complete with spurs. The image remained stationary for a few moments and then moved away. I heard footsteps receding into the distance along a wooden sidewalk. I looked up to my headboard. Sure enough, there was my familiar drip feed, so I knew I had to be in my hospital bed, but I still wasn't quite sure.

I strained to hear whatever I could in hopes of getting a clue. Again, there were footsteps on the sidewalk. More shadows passed across the window, but nothing as recognizable as the cowboy. *This must be a western town,* I thought. *Cowboy hats, spurs, wooden sidewalks — what else could it be?*

Then, I saw the cowboy again. This time he came straight into the room and closed the door behind him. He had a gruff voice and was wearing the unmistakable star-shaped badge of a sheriff. He brushed passed my bed and went to a desk at the far end of the room, where he shuffled through some papers, walked around the desk, and then sat down. Leaning backwards in the well-padded chair, he propped up his feet, lifted the brim of his hat with a quick upward flick of his thumb, and growled at me, "So I guess they left you for us to be doing the nurse-maiding."

This was not a good start.

"I have no idea," I tried to reassure him. If this were not a good plan for him, then it certainly would not be in my best interest either. "Maybe there was an emergency at the hospital, and they needed some reliable accommodation for some of us older patients. They must trust you," I mouthed; but I don't think he could lip-read.

He took a cigar from a box on the corner of the desk and carefully cut into it with his knife. He never looked in my direction, but proceeded to light up. The sheriff — and I was now convinced he was the sheriff — was soon sitting in a swirling cloud of tobacco smoke.

At that moment, someone whom I took to be his deputy burst through the door. He appeared to be extremely agitated. "You're needed right away, boss. There's been a real bad accident behind the Main Street Bank." The two of them left in a hurry.

Why would I be left in a place like this, I wondered, *where one could be alone for hours? It may be all right for someone who isn't so dependant on others for help, but certainly not for me.* I'd no sooner formed that thought when a male nurse came into the room. As he made me comfortable, I tried to use my eyes to enquire as to why I was left here; but he didn't seem to notice and was soon on his way.

The next thing I knew it was much lighter. The sun high in the sky told me I must have slept through the night and well into the next day. I heard voices. The Sheriff and his deputy were seemingly having quite a discussion. I couldn't tell if I was the subject of their sometimes-heated debate, but I hoped not. Eventually, they put on their hats and stomped out of the office.

What now? I wondered. I was starting to get quite uncomfortable and hoped my nurse, or anyone for that matter, would come along and pay some attention to me. If only they would let me know what was happening, the waiting might not be so bad.

Some time later — it seemed like hours, but was probably only thirty minutes or so — a nurse came in and started to tidy up my bed. Soon, several others came. One was wheeling a chair. *At least I am now going to get attention, and with luck, someone will take me out of this makeshift ward.*

I was wrong.

After transferring me from the bed to the chair, all the nurses, save one, left; and I was promptly wheeled through the back door. We went through a glass door and into a sort of lobby that overlooked a covered walkway on the other side of which were storerooms filled with parts for beds and chairs. I didn't remember ever having been there.

The nurse parked my wheelchair, set the brake, and uttering "I'll be back in two minutes," left me on my own again. Right! I thought. I couldn't count the number of times I had heard that before.

People were coming and going, but no one paid more than passing attention to me. By this time, I was really confused. I couldn't have been left there to enjoy the fresh air because there wasn't any. Suddenly one of my regular nurses came in pushing an empty wheelchair.

"I see you haven't gone to sleep on me," she remarked. "That's good. I have a new chair for you to try. I'll get some help and we'll transfer you."

"Great!" I exclaimed. "Tell me though, will you then take me back to my room? I feel isolated here, and certainly don't want to be left in the Sheriff's office again."

The nurse looked at me rather oddly and then a little smile crossed her face. "The sheriff's office," she said. "What do you mean? You haven't left your room since last week!"

Post Script: I suspect this was one of those days the nursing staff were trying out different sizes and styles of wheel chairs that I would fit into, without my falling out!

~ Author

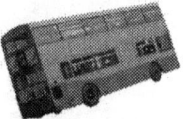

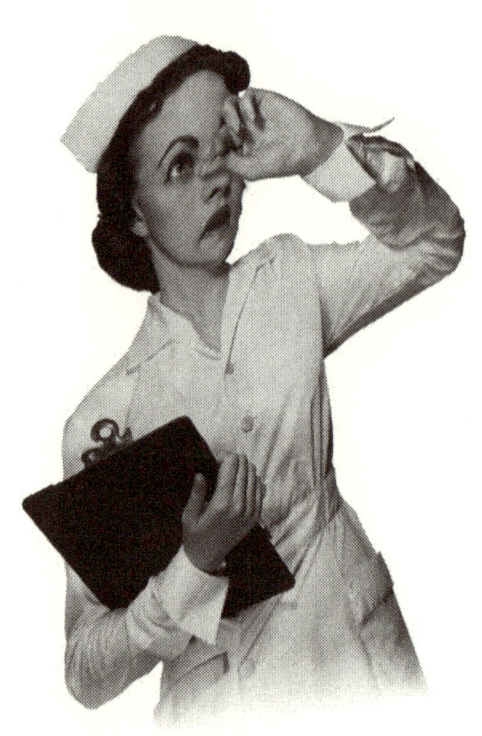

Guardian Angel in a Stetson

I awoke one morning to find an interesting looking envelope on my bed. I opened it and discovered an invitation to an open house being held the following week. Although I didn't recognize the sender or the address, I thought that I would have ample time to discover the origin of the invitation.

Sometime later, when a respiratory therapist named Don came into the room to suction me, I suddenly recalled that he'd talked about a friend who had the same name as the one on my invitation. I asked Don if he had been invited to a party, thinking this might tell me whom the invitation was from and, possibly, why I was included. He said he had been and added that the party was being given by a rather eccentric friend of his named Mike, who had a habit of throwing somewhat less than wild parties at his home in the country.

115

"I don't think I will be going, though," Don said. Then, "Don't tell me you have also had the misfortune to receive an invitation from Mike?" Obviously feeling guilty over his indiscretion, he added, "Don't take me too seriously; he's not a bad chap, really."

"Yes," I told him. "I've been invited, and I'd like to have a night out, so I think I will accept. Sure you won't change your mind and join me?" Don shook his head.

The day of the open house arrived. Since I had decided it was best not to go too early, it must have been about 8:00 or even a little later when I reached Mike's house. I cannot recall how I left the hospital, but presume I had traveled in or with my wheelchair. To my surprise, I was the first one there. Mike ushered me into to a fairly large lounge and asked me to sit down. The way the furniture had been arranged indicated that we were in for an evening of playing cards.

Before long, several other people arrived and briefly introduced themselves. One of them, Kenny, appeared to be quite the organizer and obviously knew his way around. All the other guests seemed to know each other.

By now I had sensed that this was going to be one long, boring evening. I have never enjoyed playing cards, unless it happened to be Christmas, and then I was choosy as to what was played.

Kenny made the announcement that they were going to draw straws. The person who drew the shortest one would be able to leave first, and so on. It seemed everyone accepted the situation. Kenny was not a person many argued with, at least if they were wise.

How exciting, I thought sarcastically. *I only hope I draw the shortest straw.*

Mike and Kenny went into the kitchen, no doubt to cut up the straws. Then Kenny came strutting out with his hand inside a brown paper bag. He came over to me first. "Pick a straw," he grunted, pushing the bag towards me. "Here, one of these I am holding between my fingers." He very cleverly worked it so that I was unable to ferret around for a short straw. I bit my tongue and pulled. I was not impressed. If I didn't have the longest straw, I must have been very close.

Around the room he went, offering the bag to each guest in turn. Finally, it became clear. I had, indeed, pulled the longest straw. *Great,* I thought, preparing for the longest night of my life.

It was a very long night. Eventually there were just two of us left, not including Mike and Kenny. Then there was just me. Finally, the host and his shadow went into the kitchen, and without waiting, I shouted a quick "Goodnight" and was on my way.

I had only a rough idea of where I was. South seemed to be the right direction, so that is the way I turned. It was almost dark, and I was way out in the country, so there were no streetlights, but the vague outline of trees were visible by the light of the quarter moon. Very soon, I came upon a gas station with a large convenience store attached. Being both hungry and thirsty, I wheeled in. The store was full of people—too full for this late at night—and although it was difficult to pinpoint just what, there seemed to be more going on than just the buying of cigarettes and bad coffee.

Having made my purchases, I proceeded to the checkout and was waiting my turn when suddenly there was a commotion. Several police cars with lights flashing and sirens screaming peeled into the parking lot, and soon the place was crawling with cops. The cashier urgently beckoned me over and told me it was a normal police raid that happened frequently at this time of night and that I ought not be involved. "You don't look like one of the people they're looking for," she reassured me. I took that as a compliment. She assisted me in a very hurried manner and rushed me out of the store. I was not sure what was going on, but it occurred to me that she seemed extremely relieved to get me out of there.

I had no idea how I would get back to the hospital, but then as I was wheeling down the main road, still headed south, a motor-cycle-riding respiratory therapist, complete with white coat, pulled up alongside and asked if I could use a ride. I did not hesitate for a second. The therapist, whom I now saw was not Don or anyone else I recognized, pointed to his sidecar, indicating I should get in. I later learned his name was Regan. He folded up my wheelchair and loaded it, rather precariously I thought. It didn't matter. I was happy to be getting a ride.

Off we went. It was quite exhilarating. After a few miles Regan turned to me and shouted, "I have to get gas." A station appeared at a fork in the road up ahead, and he slowed down. The night was dark, and the shadowy shapes of trees could be made out at the edge of the area penetrated by the station's lights.

We stopped at one of the pumps. Regan cut the ignition, swung his leg over the bike, turned, and went over to talk to someone. In the meantime, several police officers arrived. I imagined they were looking for me, but I had no idea why. If they were, the one thing that would surely give me away was the wheelchair. In the sidecar, I would appear to be just another ambulatory person.

Just as the officers were starting to question the staff at the far pumps, a man dressed in a dark grey cape and a black Stetson, whom I was sure I recognized, came out of the trees, walked quickly by the sidecar, calmly took my folded wheelchair, and disappeared into the darkness. It was Dwayne.[2]

How great! I thought. Thanks to him, I now had nothing that could give me away.

After a few minutes, Regan returned and started to gas up. By that time, the policemen had reached our pump. They looked briefly at me and then looked harder at the motorcycle and sidecar. Much to my relief, they noticed nothing unusual and walked by in the direction of the office.

The next morning, no one expressed surprise at seeing me back in my bed. I could hear the day nurses coming on duty, so knew it must have been around seven. For some reason, it always seemed the noisiest part of the day, and I often had the thought that the nurses were having a brief party before the night staff left.

The next night was totally different. Actually, it was late afternoon when I slipped out of my room. There was only one nurse on the desk, and her back was turned. I let myself

2 Dwayne was one of my sons in law (Author)

out through the double doors and, in a very relaxed frame of mind, made my way to the south entrance. I stepped out of the main building and went past a small residence, which housed some of the nurses and respiratory therapists. A little further on, there was a garden, complete with benches. It was shaded and inviting, and I could not resist. I selected the best seat, made myself comfortable, and enjoyed the warm air.

In the garden, I was able to contemplate what was happening to me. I knew I could not use most of my muscles, but was encouraged by the knowledge that new limbs were growing to replace ones that no longer functioned. For example, a second right shoulder was growing anew alongside the old one[3]. I could adopt the new one or keep the old one. It was a tough choice because I had no way of knowing which, in the final analysis, would function better.

I must have fallen asleep because I suddenly woke up and discovered I was being fastened to the seat with a couple of stout ropes. A man I didn't recognize was hurriedly tying the last knot and muttering something like, "You will freeze tonight." He then backed away. It was too late to struggle. In a flash, he disappeared.

Now what can I do? I wondered. *Someone will surely come by before long and untie me.*

Eventually, someone did. It was not yet dark, but was starting to get quite cool when from behind the trees appeared the now-familiar figure dressed in the long grey cape and Stetson. Again Dwayne had come to my rescue!

---

3 Just a reminder, this was a dream! (Author).

120

"Let's get you untied," he said. "Who did this any-way?" Before I even had a chance to reply, he was deftly cutting the ropes.

"Someone who intended me to freeze to death overnight," I suggested. "Or at the very least, someone who thought my muscles would stop growing as the temperature dropped." Before I could say more, Dwayne had vanished. I didn't even see him go. At that point, I really started to wonder if I had imagined him. However it had happened, though, I was free to move around.

By that time, it was getting decidedly cooler, and I decided to go back to the hospital. As I passed the nurse's residence, one of my nurses named Penelope was returning from her shift. "You look cold," she remarked with a con-cerned look. "You had better come in, and warm up."

Once inside, I found a place close to a very inviting, but rather neglected fire, put my feet up, and closed my eyes.

How does Dwayne always manage to be at the right place at the right time? I wondered.

Post Script: Why in a Stetson? I am not sure. I have not even seen Dwayne wear a cowboy hat. Some may say that's unusual for Calgary, the home of the Calgary Stampede!

~ Author

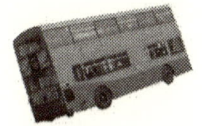

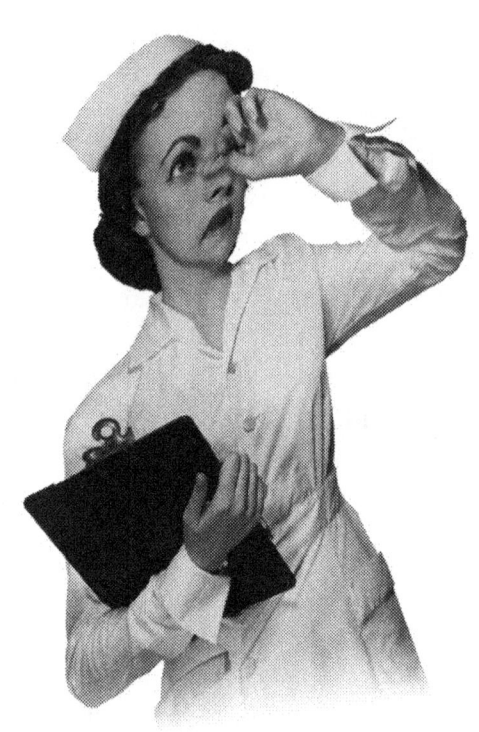

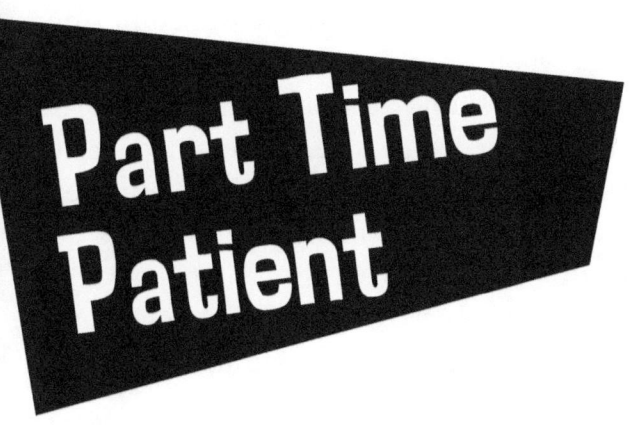

Part Time Patient

I couldn't decide whether I was a hospital patient or not. I knew, however, that I was overseas.

In the daytime I was able to go anywhere I wished, either by car or on foot. It was odd, since although I knew in my inner being that I was in the hospital, no one seemed to miss me. It seemed I didn't spend much time there at all.

The hospital was on an island that used to be a British Colony. There was a small city close by, and I seemed to spend a lot of time near its harbour. I also spent a great deal of time at the Harbour Cliff Hotel, which was just off the road leading to the water. I always tried to make it there for lunch, since they served up good food and were not too expensive.

The evenings were a different matter. The hotel was extremely crowded, and it was difficult to get any attention, particularly for me as I had trouble getting around. However, this evening was to be different.

I had just left the car and was crossing the road in front of the Harbour Cliff when I heard what the familiar sound of musical car horns.[4] The sound was so distinctive that you just couldn't miss it. I turned and smiled. It reminded me of home. Just before we left, these horns were becoming very popular. Now, they were obviously being sold here.

Continuing towards the entrance, I checked in my pocket for my wallet, pushed against the revolving doors, and immediately found myself in a mass of humanity. People were milling around everywhere.

I had been here often enough to know my way around and made straight for the lower floor, which was a favourite of the locals. It was more crowded than it had ever been before. With difficulty, I made my way to a table, sat down in the only vacant seat, and waited for the server. It was then that I spotted two women who I thought looked familiar. One of them had seen me, too and was waving in recognition.

I decided to try to join them. *Try* was the operative word, since I was having a tough time moving my legs.

Finally, after much struggling, I reached the ladies' table. Now I saw they were two of my nurses, Colette and Patricia. They made room, then proceeded to scold me for being there.

"You should not be out of the hospital," Patricia remonstrated. "Why do you do it?"

---

4 I later discovered the 'musical car horns' were not what they seemed. They were, in fact, the sounds of the alarm on my ventilator, indicating a problem

Part Time Patient

"Nothing ever happens in the day-time, and no one ever misses me, so why shouldn't I do some exploring?" I reasoned. "I can't just sit around doing nothing—but, please don't mention this to the patient-care manager or the doctors."

"Brian," Colette said with deliberate emphasis. "What are we going to do with you?" They both laughed, obviously realizing it was hopeless to try and talk me out of my exploits.

"Let me buy you a drink," I suggested, hoping it would divert them from this subject.

"How are you getting back to the hospital?" Patricia asked.

"I am not really sure," I responded. "Usually a respiratory therapist picks me up in one of their trucks. They seem to know where I will be at any given time. There is probably one waiting outside for me right now."

At that moment, Patricia's husband, Desmond, showed up. He was the designated driver, it seemed, and his arrival was the signal that it was time to leave. Colette turned to me, and suggested I go with them. "If your R. T. truck is waiting for you," she said with a big smile, "that's fine; but if not, you are coming with us. We are not leaving you here." I agreed. To argue would have been pointless. We made our way to the lobby and out the revolving doors.

There was no large white truck to be seen anywhere. I was disappointed. I knew my companions had not believed me, and I wanted to demonstrate that I was not imagining that the respiratory therapists provided transportation for me. Colette looked knowingly in my direction. "I don't see anyone waiting for you," she teased, as we proceeded towards Desmond's car.

Desmond helped me get in, and we were on our way to an apartment the three of them shared — because of the cost Colette later explained. I must have been lulled to sleep by the smooth ride because, the next thing I knew, we had arrived at our destination.

Once inside the very comfortable apartment, hot coffee was the order of the day. After sitting around talking enjoying the warm glow of a log fire, Desmond turned to Patricia and explained he was on an early shift the next day. "We had better take our leave of these two, and get moving," he added.

"Sure," Patricia responded. "I have an early start too. 'Night guys. See you whenever."

It was then that it dawned on me I had gone to the Harbour Cliff Hotel in my car. It was, however, too late to do anything about it, since Desmond would not appreciate having to get out of bed and run me back for it. *Oh well, I will just have to pick it up tomorrow,* I thought.

"Brian, you look miles away," Colette remarked, as she finished tidying up the room.

"Sorry," I replied, rather lamely. "You guys have been so kind. I think the warmth from the fire has gotten to me." She was making herself comfortable on the rug and gazing into the hearth. She looked very thoughtful for a moment, then turned to me and posed the question, "Are you interested in history?" She sure knew how to get my attention. History and politics were among my favourite subjects.

"Yes, indeed," I told her. "And I presume from the question that you are, also. Do you have a favourite period?"

Once on that topic of mutual interest, we covered everything from the Black Death in the Middle Ages to English Kings and Queens up to the reign of Victoria. Time passed so quickly, and it must have been well after two a.m. when the doorbell rang. Colette jumped up, peeked out the window and, upon recognizing the visitor, opened the door. I could tell from the guest's distinctive voice that it was Clint, the respiratory therapist.

"I am here to give Brian a ride," he said.

"How did you know he was here?" she asked.

"That was easy," he responded, smiling. "One of the other respiratory therapists saw him leaving the Harbour Cliff with you guys. We all know he's a late-nighter!"

"Well, I guess we have to call it a day," I said, turning to the good-natured Colette. "Thanks for your hospitality. I hope I haven't kept you up too late." I gripped her hand as a thank-you gesture. She responded with a gentle kiss on my cheek.

"Good night, Brian. You get yourself safely back to the hospital."

With that, Clint and I left to get into the white R.T. truck, and as we did, he gave me a broad grin. "Nice lady!"

Post Script: For the first weeks and months into my time of hospitalisation, it was difficult to believe I was in hospital full time. I seemed to know I was supposed to be there some of the time, like overnight, but nothing ever seemed to be happening, no tests, no treatments, nothing. No one seemed to miss me

A Dream IMPOSSIBLE

when I imagined myself wandering at will, during the day, surprisingly, enjoying full mobility, most of the time.

~ Author

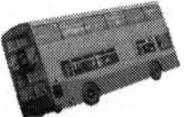

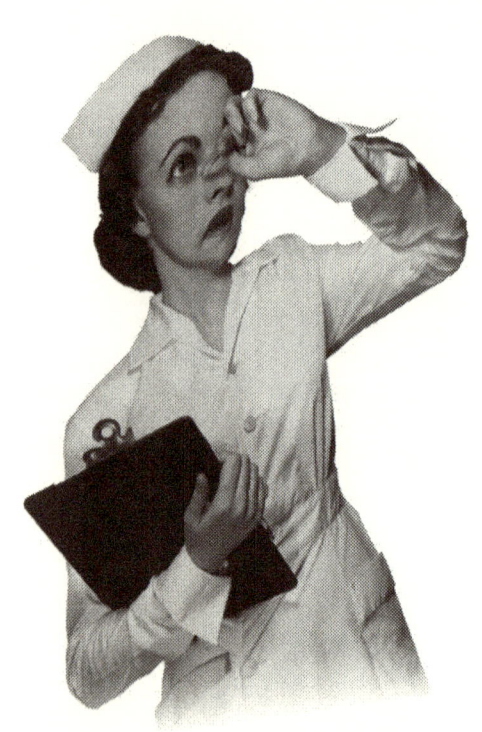

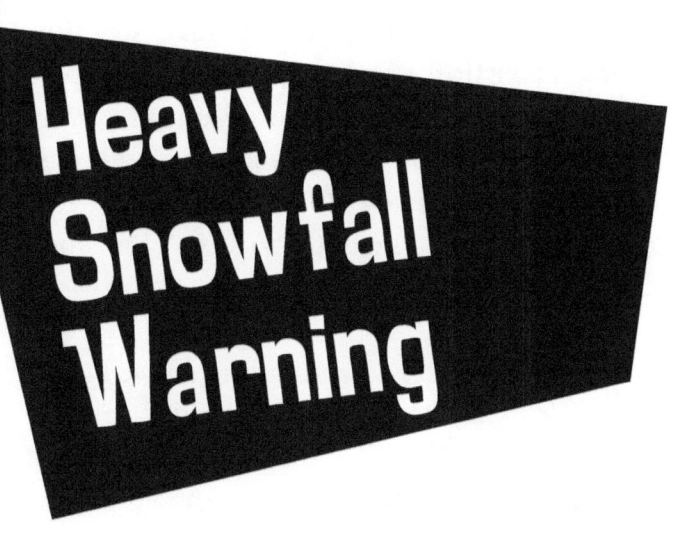

Heavy Snowfall Warning

Here I was downtown, but in my hospital bed with my oxygen and intravenous feeding equipment hanging from the headboard. It was four in the afternoon, and I was hoping to get a lift back to the hospital. The traveling respiratory therapists (RT's) had arranged to meet me at the corner of Fourth and Fourth, where I had just arrived. It was starting to snow. To pass some time, I traveled farther down the block to Radio Hut and spent a little time window shopping and watching a show on their large-screen TV.

I was about to leave when the program changed and a heavy snowfall warning flashed across the screen. The programming then returned to normal, but I realized I did not know which areas were affected by the warning or even if my city, Calgary, was included, so I decided to stay a little longer, hoping for a repeat. I didn't have to wait long. Yes, the warning was intended for Calgary, so I now paid a lot more attention. It seemed very serious. Commuters and others in the downtown area were advised not to leave, but to find accommodation wherever they found themselves. At least 25 cm. of snow were expected, along with extremely high winds. That spelt blizzard conditions.

Just my luck! I thought. *How could I arrange accommodations that would be accessible in my hospital bed?* I decided to make my way back to the corner of Fourth and Fourth in hopes that my RT friends would show up. By now it was snowing heavily, and my pillows and blankets were getting covered, so to stay dry, I had to keep my head well down under the covers. *This is no good,* I thought. *I had better try to make for Woodson's and get some shelter.*

I can't remember where I parked my bed, but I do remember being on a shuttle bus looking over the driver's shoulder and seeing what was perhaps the worst winter weather I had ever witnessed. It was a complete whiteout. The snow was falling so heavily, it was virtually impossible to see anything. After we had gone a few blocks, the driver turned to me and asked which of Woodson's entrances I needed. I marvelled at the fact that he could identify a particular entrance through the blinding snow.

"It doesn't matter," I responded. "Just drop me where you can."

Once inside store, I made my way to the central escalator and proceeded to the top floor. As I reached the third floor, I was pleasantly surprised to see Ken Waterton, one of my colleagues from the office. It was natural that the weather would be the first topic of conversation.

"If this continues, I guess we are both here for the night," I commented. There was no sign of it abating.

"I think you're right. Have you ever used the Woodson Club when you were stuck downtown overnight?" he asked.

I was rather confused by the question and said quite truthfully that I had not. I didn't even know that the Woodson Club existed. I had thought I'd just make myself comfortable between a couple of counters, using my rather generously sized parka as a blanket. I liked Ken's idea better. "Okay," he said. "Why don't we go to the restaurant on the top floor, get some food, and afterwards we can go to the Club and I will introduce you. You will be more comfortable there."

"Sounds good to me," I replied.

Over supper, I quizzed him about the Woodson Club. Apparently it cost two hundred dollars to get in; but he explained that there was an outside overhead rail system, which ran from the top floor, and if we climbed onto one of the railcars at mid-floor, we could get in free.

"I don't understand, " I said. "Is there no other way in? How does this rail system work?"

"Well, there is if you want to pay $200," he explained. "The outside rail system is a one way downhill track around the perimeter of the building. It serves as an alternative to elevators to reach certain floors including high security areas, and will suit us just fine.

"I know what your next question will be," he continued. You want to know how we enter the system at mid-floor? After we've had supper, I will demonstrate. It's quite easy. We do have to act quickly, though, as you will see. Basically at each mid-floor point there is a turnout from the main track, and usually a spare railcar is parked there. The trick is to apply the brakes so that the railcar coming down stops just past the turnout. We then have to reroute the track to allow the railcar to run downhill and connect up with the main train. This is all run by computer, so after being braked between floors, the car only stops for sixty seconds, and then automatically restarts; but it's enough time for us to hop in."

"Sounds dangerous," I said. "You do seem to be familiar with the whole operation, though. So let's say I'm game."

I wondered later how the railcars running from the top and then circling around the building down to the basement ever got back up to where they started.

After finishing supper we decided to have a couple of drinks while contemplating Ken's plan for hitching a ride on the railcar system. I asked how we could get to the rail track in between this and the lower floor. He indicated by a casual gesture that we could gain access through the fire exit door just behind us. All we had to do was make this look very innocent and not attract any attention.

"Let's go now," he said abruptly, "while there are not to many people around."

With that, we drank up and slipped through the fire exit. There was a flight of stairs, and at the halfway point there was a doorway, which we entered. Ken seemed a bit hesitant, but upon hearing railcar traffic around the next corner, he said he guessed we were headed in the right direction. Sure enough, we came upon a spare railcar just where we expected to find it. Taking my lead from Ken, I set the trackside brake, returned to the railcar, and jumped in as he went for the handbrake. Now all we had to do was wait for the next train.

We didn't have long to wait. Moments later a three-car train was brought to a halt by the brake we had set. By now, high winds were blowing snow over us, making the footing rather treacherous. I was very aware of the abyss below.

We had to move fast since the train was almost stopped. Ken released the brake, and I jumped out to change the turnout switch, hopping back in just in time. In the meantime, Ken had jumped out and connected our car to the main train. He was also just in time, and soon the whole train, including our car, was gaining speed. Twice, we were stopped by people joining the train the same way we had.

"Which floor are we making for Ken?"

"The second," he said. "It's the only way into the club!"

As he made his comment, we reached our destination. We were now able to mingle with the fare-paying passengers, as tickets no longer had to be shown. That made me feel a lot better.

The club entrance was nothing spectacular, just old-fashioned double swinging doors with an attendant behind a desk just inside. Ken introduced me and showed his pass, which allowed access for him and a guest. We passed through the lobby and entered a rather large hall. At this point Ken pointed to a pile of blankets and pillows in the middle of the floor and suggested that I help myself and find a spot to bed down for the night. Then he turned and left.

I saw one or two people I recognized from the hospital, and they acknowledged me as I went by. I grabbed some blankets and looked for a place to settle in. Many people had obviously arrived earlier than Ken and I, so space was at a premium. I noticed that most had paired off and had a momentary pang about being alone.

On finding a gap, I bedded down and prepared to go to sleep for the night feeling thankful that I had shelter and wasn't stranded outside in the blizzard. Just as I was about to doze off, who should walk through the door but Clarisa, one of my nurses! She recognized me immediately and waved. I couldn't help feeling flattered. She was a very caring nurse and a very attractive young lady.

I didn't expect that Clarisa and her companion — whom I thought I recognized as another nurse — would want to talk to me. She appeared to know some of the people and chatted with several acquaintances as she made her way to a group in the far corner. After what seemed to be a brief conversation, though, Clarisa left the group and came in my direction.

"Hi Brian," she greeted me, "could I ask you a favour?"

"Of course." I replied. "How can I help?"

"I'm not sure that I'm too comfortable here. The group in the corner is expecting me to stay with them, and quite frankly, I don't wish to. Can I tell them that you have invited me to share your blanket?"

"Sure, no problem."

With that, she placed her drawstring bag down beside my pillow, thanked me, and said she would be back in a few minutes. Ironically, 'Back in a few minutes' is what all the nurses say all the time!

True to her word, this time, she in fact was back in a few minutes. Her nursing instincts appeared to take over, and she asked how my feet were. Any Guillain-Barré patient will appreciate the importance of that enquiry, because if the feet are comfortable, it is likely that the patient is comfortable, overall.

"They're sort of okay." I replied. "They do have a restless feeling though."

Clarisa responded by uncovering my feet and giving them a gentle massage. Anything less than gentle could prove extremely painful.

After a short time, she finished her massage, took off her shoes and street clothes, and went to the blanket storage area in the middle of the hall for a thicker blanket. She was concerned that I was sleeping directly on the floor. After rolling me over on my side and sliding the new blanket under me, she returned me to my original position and then felt my forehead as though to check out my temperature, and continued stroking my brow.

I was always putty in the hands of anyone who ran fingers through my hair or did anything pleasant to my head. I even loved having my hair washed or getting a haircut. I found Clarisa's touch very soothing.

All good things come to an end, however, and after a while she stood back and said, "It's bedtime, Brian." With that, she reached across for the edge of my blanket and slipped under it. After giving me a hug, she turned her back to me, snuggled up close, pulled my arms around her, and that's how we went to sleep.

After a couple of hours, I awoke, tried to rise up on my elbows, intending to gently kiss Clarisa's cheek, but could not. She must have awoken at the same time and realized what I was trying to do because she raised her cheek towards me, accepting my gesture. Then we slept again, and that is all I remember.

The next morning I found myself in my hospital bed in the same intensive care room that I had occupied for some time. Sure enough, I could hear the regular 'clip clop, clip clop' of my ventilator, and I gained comfort from that and the sight of my intravenous drip-feed equipment. I didn't have to worry about the retrieval of my hospital bed parked somewhere downtown...probably covered with two feet of snow!

But wait! I thought to myself. *If my hospital bed is still parked somewhere downtown, whose bed am I in now? And how on earth did I get back here?*

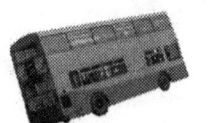

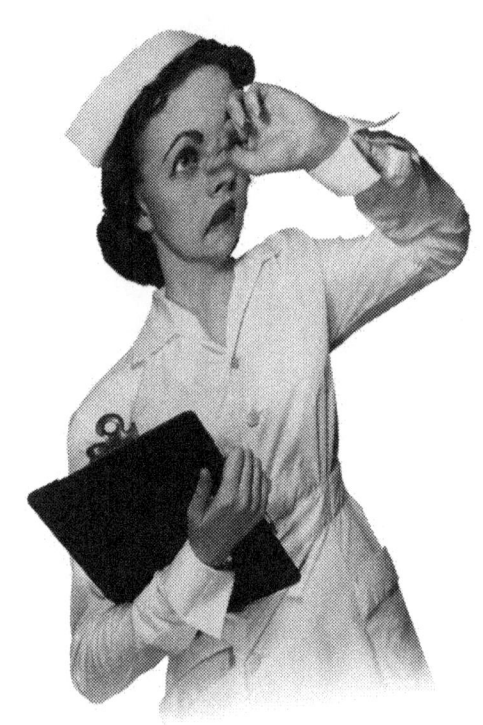

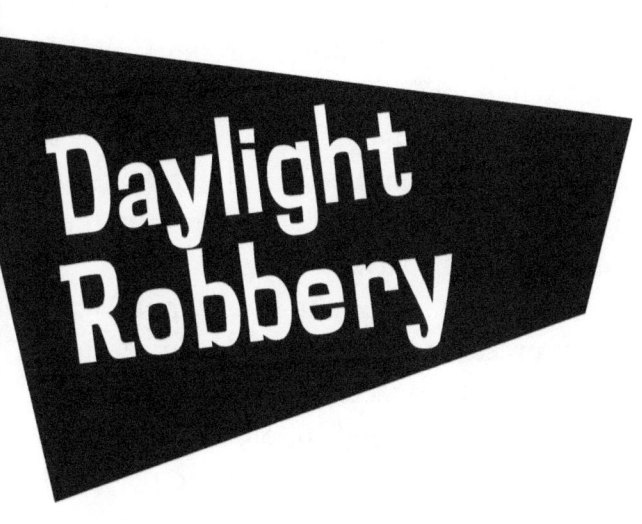

Daylight Robbery

For some reason, I liked to window shop in one particular small hobby and craft store, but never spent any money there. Others also must have done more looking than buying because there were notices that the store was closing down. This made me sad. I had spent many grey winter afternoons there happily browsing.

I wondered if someone else would take it over or if maybe the place would be gutted. Nothing stays the same forever.

Very soon my questions were answered. There was good news and there was bad news. The bad news was that a retired army colonel with a reputation for being unethical and taking advantage of others had announced his intention to purchase the business. The good news was that he apparently planned to continue running it as a hobby and crafts store.

One item in the store that had always fascinated me was a special sort of modelling clay. At normal room temperature, it was stiff, but when warmed up through being handled, it would become soft and pliable. It was used mainly to make scale models of finely detailed buildings, exterior fences, and walls. There were models of buildings sculpted and moulded by the staff on display.

Some time passed before I visited the shop again. When the next opportunity presented itself, I could sense many changes. For one thing, I was conscious of being under surveillance from the moment I walked in. *So, this is how the new owner is going to operate,* I thought. After a quick walk through, I decided enough was enough. It just wasn't the same store, so I left.

I couldn't keep away for long, though. I was fascinated by the possibilities offered by that modelling clay; so a few days later, I decided to go back and buy a few dollars worth. When I arrived, I saw the new owner had raised the prices substantially; and there was also a notice warning shoppers that they would be required to purchase the product if, in handling it, they altered the shape or form of the product. As on the last visit, it was soon obvious I was under surveillance. That made me very angry and I became determined to fight back.

As I handled the clay models, I was careful not to change their shape — something that could happen just from the heat of one's hand. A large woman, whom I suspected was the store detective, watched every move I made. She appeared to be known to a number of the shoppers. Even when she stopped to talk to someone else, she kept her eyes on me. To make life difficult for her, I would turn away and, when I was done with an item, I'd put it down outside her line of sight. That would drive her crazy! This cat and mouse game continued for most of the afternoon. I was determined not to be outdone, but I think she had other ideas.

A short while later, the new owner made his entrance. He went straight over to the store detective, and the two of them went into a huddle. It didn't surprise me to see them looking and pointing from time to time in my direction. I was sure the heat would now be on me, but in what way, I could never have guessed.

It was getting near closing time when I took a last look at the clay models. I picked up a model of a bungalow and spent a little time admiring the detail inside. I was too engrossed to notice the detective crank up the heat. As it turned out, I was standing right under a duct and, all of a sudden, it was getting very warm. I loosened my collar, and then became aware that the clay model I was holding was starting to get really soft, and indentations were appearing in the clay where my palm and fingers came in contact with it. The harder I tried to smooth it out, the more of a mess I made.

"That will be $175, please." A sales assistant had moved up behind me and obviously decided I'd changed the appearance of the model and would have to pay for it. "Please take it to the check-out and settle up there," she continued.

What an underhanded way to get me to buy something. I

decided that to sink that low, they must have been pretty desperate for income. There was no doubt the product had been changed somewhat, but that would not have happened had they not deliberately turned up the heat.

At that point, my wife came in looking for a ride home. I explained what had happened, and we were in total agreement as to how we should handle this situation. I replaced the model, turned to the sales assistant, and asked her to accompany us to the checkout. After complaining about the way I had been tricked, I assured the cashier and sales assistant that I would accept some responsibility and consider a reasonable claim, but refused to pay in full for the item I had allegedly damaged.

"Then we shall have to charge you with shoplifting," asserted the store detective, who had joined the group.

"Sorry," I responded. "Not only am I taking nothing out of the shop, I am inviting you to submit a claim, which, if reasonable, will be accepted. Here is my address. That cannot be called shoplifting by anyone's definition."

The response from the store detective was rather predictable. "The new owner would not agree," he said emphatically. "He has a very aggressive policy regarding losses of any kind; and it is my duty to implement that policy. If you don't pay up, you will be arrested the moment you leave the shop. We have already called the police." I turned to my wife and suggested we withdraw to the back of the store and discuss the situation further.

As soon as we were out of sight, we went through a doorway leading to some stairs. They led into a large storage area, where we proceeded to hide among all the packages, cartons, and supplies. On the way up I opened a window to make it appear we had made our escape that way. It must have worked because the subsequent search of the storage area was very perfunctory.

After waiting for things to settle down, we decided to climb out of the open window and make our way to the car under the cover of darkness. To our dismay, when we reached the window and leaned out to make sure the coast was clear, we saw the flashing lights of two police cars. They must have known we were still there and were waiting for us to come out. This called for a different plan. We climbed out of the window, keeping as low a profile as possible. Instead of making for the car, we went the opposite way into a wooded area and made our way through the trees to the main road. Then we walked home.

The next morning I awoke in need of a suction. The day nurse came in to check me out and promised to call a respiratory therapist. While awaiting relief, I couldn't help wondering how long it would be before the craft and hobby store filed a claim. This worried me somewhat, although I knew they would not succeed in a charge of shoplifting. Still, I was dealing with someone who was unscrupulous, so I imagined anything could happen.

Days later, my wife came in on her daily visit and held out a letter from the hobby store. It was a claim for $750! "That is outrageous," I told Sylvia. Could you reply for me? Tell them, under the circumstances, we make a counter offer of $75, which will be withdrawn if not accepted within thirty days. Even that is being more generous than they deserve."

We never heard anything further on the subject. No wonder, really. A few months later, I came to the realization there was no hobby shop or any other store in the place I had imagined it.

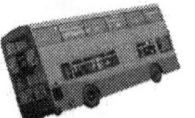

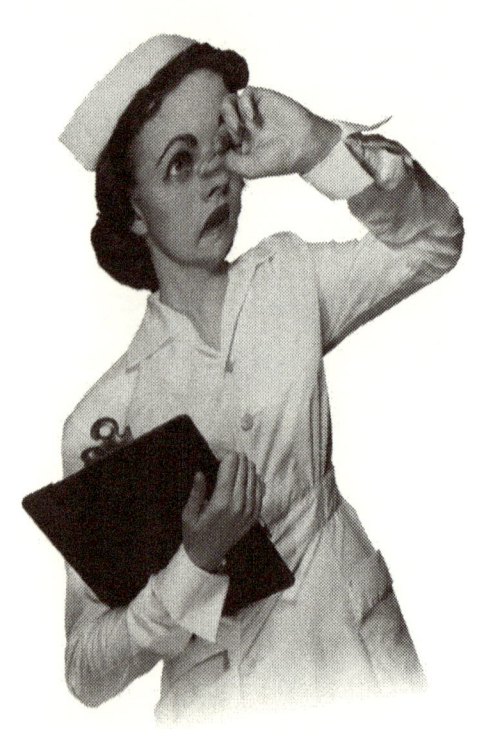

Who Wants to Buy a Double-Decker Bus ?

It can be hot in Calgary in July, and this day was. Not yet eight in the morning, and it was already twenty-three degrees Centigrade. I'd just dropped Sylvia off to meet her friends and was driving with the windows down, enjoying the warm fresh air. I was in a part of the city that I wasn't familiar with, and when I noticed a turn leading to the foot of a gorge, I thought I would explore. After about a kilometre or so, the road started to rise quite steeply.

Now I was climbing to the top of the gorge. Suddenly, after rounding a tight bend, I saw a large notice at the side of the road: "Win $50,000 by having your car driven over the gorge at the lowest possible speed!" was the message. "Lose, and we take your car in exchange for a trade-in."

This sounded tempting. According to the notice, the lowest speed achieved so far was ten kilometres per hour.

The camber of the road on the bridge was such that if a car actually stopped, it would surely fall off. For some reason, though, I was convinced that I could drive over it at seven kilometres per hour without taking a tumble. It would be close, but I could do it.

I pulled over when I saw a small wooden cabin with same 'Win $50,000...' poster. A young man was standing at the door. *Probably a summer student,* I thought. Upon getting closer, I decided he looked familiar. Then I was sure. "Your mother is a nurse at the hospital, isn't she?" I asked. He nodded. Now I knew I would get a fair deal here.

"All right, I'll buy a ticket and drive over," I asserted. "How much?"

"Just ten dollars" was his reply.

I paid him and looked to the gate, expecting it to be opened for me. Instead, the young man held out his hand and asked for my keys. My stomach tightened. "Why?" I asked.

"I have to drive you over. Those are the rules." Now I saw I had neglected to read the small print. What do I do now? I thought. I decided it was still a good deal. I didn't think the nurse's son would take unfair advantage, at least I hoped he wouldn't. When he agreed that I could ride with him, I gave him the keys and told him I was sure that it was possible to drive this car over the bridge at seven kilometres per hour. He nodded. Then, knowing I was beyond the point of no return, I moved over to the passenger side and relaxed.

Off we went. As we approached the bridge, we slowed down to about fifteen kilometres per hour and, to my dismay, continued across at that speed. "What do you think you're doing?" I yelled. "You aren't even trying! You can go much slower than this."

"Sorry" was all he would say!

Now I was getting quite angry. I knew I'd been taken for a ride in more ways than one, and I was beginning to feel very foolish. *How could I get taken in like this?* I asked myself.

We quickly reached the other side, where there was another small cabin attended by four men. One appeared to be a regular employee, but the others could easily have qualified as nightclub bouncers. Had I decided to dispute the result of this "slowest over the bridge" competition, there was no doubt in my mind as to who would win the argument.

"Your keys please."

My heart sank. The man I thought to be an employee handed me a document to sign. He explained it was required by the government to confirm both the sale of my car and the fact that I was trading it in 'voluntarily'! It was becoming very clear that there would be no getting out of this. The other three men — the muscle-bound ones — had moved to block my only means of escape. The alternative was a three hundred foot drop.

I signed his waiver and looked at the receipt he handed me. I'd estimated the value of my car to be about $17,000. The receipt showed a value of $14,000, for which I would receive two trade-ins. One was a four-year-old import, dusty green, ill-kept and rusted, worth $6,000. The other, which I'd be told about later, was valued at $8,000.

I didn't believe how stupid I'd been! How could I tell Sylvia and my daughters that I'd gambled away our virtually new car? How could I admit to behaving so recklessly? And it wasn't only my family. What about the bank? I still owed money on that car. Not much admittedly, but the fact remained that there was a lien on it.

The next morning I awoke in the Intensive Care Unit, still connected to a ventilator and an intravenous drip feed. Nurses came and went, as did breakfast time and bath time. Or was it the other way around? I wasn't sure and could not have cared less. My problem was how to tell the bank manager!

Two days went by. Then one of the respiratory therapists came into my room and gave me a cheque for $4,000 dollars and a promissory note for, of all things, a Double-Decker bus. I was considering what it might mean as he gave me one of my regular suctions. *What was his part in this,* I wondered? And what could I do with a Double-Decker? I still had not phoned the bank, and this was worrying me more than anything else.

I spent all the next day trying to figure out how to phone the bank manager and what the consequences of that conversation might be. Since I couldn't use my hands, someone would have to dial and hold the phone for me, and that could only happen if a telephone were brought into my room in Intensive Care. That created another problem. Whoever held the phone could not avoid overhearing how foolish I had been. What a dilemma!

The following day brought more problems. After what would have been breakfast time for most people, but not me since I was on intravenous feeding, I happened to look out of my window. It was a beautiful sunny day with typical Alberta blue skies. Then I saw something that changed my day. A red Double-Decker bus — my Double-Decker bus — was parked on the road outside the hospital. I did not need this. Looking around, I could see the nurses were all occupied, so out of bed I leapt and hurried out of the hospital, hoping I wouldn't be missed. I ran right into the arms of the respiratory therapist who had brought me the money.

"I was hoping to see you," he said. "Here are the keys for your bus!"

Hardly pausing, I took them and continued out of the building. I had never driven a bus before, so things in the next little while could prove to be tricky.

Seeing the bus at close quarters brought all the earlier concerns rushing back to mind. I couldn't keep it, that much was clear; but how could it be disposed of? In the meantime it couldn't be left where it was because it was in a no parking zone. Then I had an idea. I had a friend who ran a small business in a subdivision of Calgary, and I thought perhaps he might have space for me to park the bus until I could decide what to do with it. *It's worth a try!* I thought.

I struggled into the drivers seat, made myself comfortable, and with some trepidation, turned the key. The engine roared to life. *Now to get this behemoth to my friend's in one piece!*

After a white-knuckled drive that took about thirty minutes, I arrived at my intended destination and swung the bus off the road onto my friend's unpaved forecourt, hitting a few potholes, which bounced the tall vehicle rather precariously from side to side, before coming to a halt. With relief, I wiped the perspiration off my forehead.

The feeling was short lived. Looking around, I failed to see any sign of activity. It appeared my friend had gone out of business or moved. Now what to do? I dared not leave the bus. What would happen if a construction crew were slated to start work here in the morning? I felt I had no option but to search around for a suitable road on which to park and just hope I could find someone in the next day or so who wanted to buy my bus.

I released the parking brake and carefully drove back to the road. After a few blocks, I noticed a rather wide road running off to the right. *Maybe this will do* I thought and signalled to make the turn. The road went uphill for a short distance, and although a number of cars were parked along it, there appeared to be a lot of space on the crest. Choosing my spot, I parallel parked the bus, set the brake, switched off the engine, and pocketed the keys.

After looking around to see if I were being observed — who would want a Double Decker parked in front of their house? — I made a quick exit, crossed over to the other sidewalk, and walked away.

It was time for my blanket bath. I had just woken up. Who had helped me back to Intensive Care and how? The hospital was a long way from where I left the bus. For a short time, my attention was held by what was happening in my room. Aides were changing the beds and one offered me a hot blanket, which I gladly accepted. No one seemed to have missed me yesterday. As soon as I was alone, my thoughts returned to selling the bus. I still had not phoned the bank!

The best way to handle a problem like this, I told myself, *is to do something about it.* The next time one of my daughters came in, I would ask her to pick up an 'Auto-Trader' publication and would use it to identify possible markets for the Double-Decker. This thought put my mind at ease. I could phone the bank later.

Several days later, my eldest daughter brought me the publication, which I gratefully put on my bedside table. This part was real. Several months later when we were reminiscing, she told me she had assumed I was looking at mini-vans capable of carrying a wheelchair.

After the visit, I asked the next nurse to come into my room if she would just flip through the magazine for me since I could not use my hands. After transferring me into the wheelchair with the help of five other nurses, she went through the book with me. To my dismay, there was absolutely nothing about any kind of bus, never mind a Double-Decker. Now I was starting to worry again. Time was passing, and I could imagine the parking tickets piling up.

I had to talk to the respiratory therapist who gave me the cheque and promissory note. "I need a suction," I told the nurse, hoping the right therapist would respond. I was disappointed. I had to wait two more days. When he finally came, I plucked up the courage to ask, "Could you help me sell the Double Decker that was traded to me? I have no contacts, but I assume you must have"

The respiratory therapist gave me a very strange look and, after a moment or two, took a step backwards and said,

"Let's talk about that tomorrow." I was puzzled by his reaction. He seemed to want to wash his hands of the matter. The next few days of worrying about accumulating parking tickets, how to contact the bank, and whom to tell, passed very slowly. Visitors came and went, and to some extent they took my mind off my concerns. My wife was a constant companion, and I appreciated being distracted from the vehicle problems.

A day or two later, my daughter Sally happened to make a very significant comment. She and her husband were keeping their M.G. in our garage. The subject came up, and I asked her if it were now easier to move in the garage than it used to be. She looked a little quizzical, but assured me there was no problem with space. I pressed further and asked what she thought about the dirty, rusted old car I now had.

"Dad, your car isn't rusty," she said. "Admittedly it's quite dusty, but then it hasn't been used for some time. You can still see the colour of it, though. The green finish still looks good."

All of a sudden things came clear. Sally was, if I dared believe her, describing my car. If my car was still at home, then I couldn't have lost it in a stupid wager. More than that, if there had been no wager, then there couldn't have been any trades either! If there were no trades, then there was no bus and no horrendous quantity of parking tickets. I had been worrying for nothing.

My car was an Eagle Vision. Just to be really sure, I

threw caution to the winds and asked Sally one more question. "What car are you referring to?"

"Your Eagle Vision, Dad. Why?"

Post Script: Why a double-decker Bus? One reason, perhaps, I have travelled many miles by double-decker bus. They were the main form of transportation in the England I knew in my younger days, but not so in North America. Disposing of one such vehicle in Canada would understandably represent an almost impossible task, adding to my level of frustration and stress.

~ Author

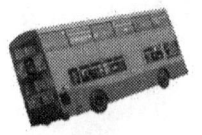

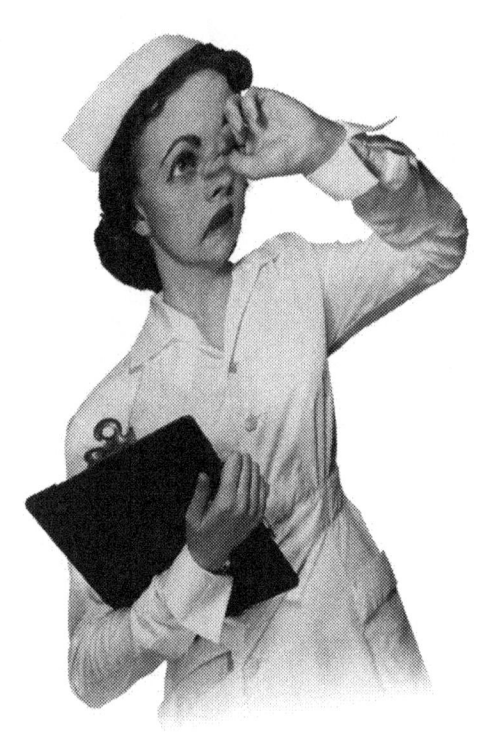

Across The Great Lake

I needed the treatment, so I had to travel. It was going to be very risky, yet I could not delay. My pneumonia was very much in evidence, and to get help, I had to take a boat across the Great Lake to Blueport, a small fishing town with a population of about ten thousand. I would have to arrange for someone to drive me to the harbour and help me onto the ferry. Luckily, there was no shortage of volunteers.

By the next morning, all necessary arrangements had been made, my ticket had been delivered, and Peter, one of the people I had been staying with, had offered to drive me to the dock. It must have been at least minus 5 degrees Centigrade — forty below if you considered the wind-chill factor. Peter pulled up as close to the boarding ramp as he could and, struggling through a fresh fall of snow, helped me to board. He wished me a safe journey and was on his way. In the hold, it was a little warmer, but not much.

The ferry was an unusual craft, almost circular, rather like a saucer. The accommodations were quite primitive. The passengers made a large circle, some sitting on sleeping bags, some lying down to keep warm, and others perched with their backs to a circular wall. I took the sleeping bag I'd been given, put it close to the wall, and just about collapsed onto it. It was so cold I could see my breath. Finally, the loading hatch was closed, and that helped me to feel a little warmer.

After perhaps a half an hour, we were moving. The lake was calm, and as we sailed through the harbour, there was just a gentle swell accompanied by the rhythmic hum of the engines.

There was a much larger contingent of First Nations people on board than I expected. One young lady was eyeing me with concern. She seemed to know I had a temperature, and after some time had elapsed, she came over, pulled my blanket more securely around me, and asked if there was anything she could do to help.

"You have chest pains?" she queried.

She didn't wait for me to answer. Seeing the sweat pouring from my brow, she indicated she would be straight back with a vapour rub. Within five minutes, she came back carrying a jar and a piece of cloth. She bared my chest and started to apply the jar's contents, rubbing with vigour.

"Why are you visiting our village at Thunder Mountain?" she asked. "We have no hospitals there, and you are in need of some care."

160

By then, I was feeling really ill. "I can get medical attention when we reach Blueport," I muttered.

"But we're not going anywhere near Blueport," she said sounding startled. We're going to Leatherhead, a small village at the foot of Thunder Mountain. You must have gotten on the wrong ferry."

That was the last thing I needed to hear. For the first time, I wondered if I were going to beat this infection. I was banking on getting treatment when the ferry docked. Now it appeared I would be ending that journey hundreds of miles from any sort of hospital or care facility.

"Don't worry," she said when she saw my reaction. "I am sure some of the elders will take you under their wing. I will talk to Chief Running Waters. He is a very compassionate man and will not want to see you in distress. He is actually travelling with us, sitting on the far side of the boat."

Hearing that relieved me some, and I summoned up a little more energy to ask the caring young lady her name. "Marina," was her reply. "I am travelling with my mother. We are returning from a shopping expedition for supplies to see us through the winter. The lake will soon be frozen over—in fact it is close to being frozen right now. If you listen, from time to time, you can hear the ice crack."

"Does that mean I am going to be stuck in Leatherhead?" My anxiety was clearly evident in my voice.

Weighing her thoughts carefully before responding, she quietly gave me encouragement. "Not really. If the Lake does freeze up—and it may not for another week or so — there would be emergency flights out to Blueport. In any case, my people will not see you alone and vulnerable." She gently wiped my forehead, and I fell asleep.

I am not sure how much later I awoke, but Marina's mother had my head cradled into her lap. I was very ill. I could sense we were nearing our destination, but had no idea how I was going to get off the ferry or where I would go. I was grateful to Marina and her mother for their attention and gained comfort from the fact that they had, apparently, taken control of my situation. I remember feeling a brief flash of concern when I heard someone say that it was so cold, it would be a miracle if I survived the crisis on this boat. Then I fell asleep again.

Suddenly, I heard chains banging against the side of the ferry and knew we must be docking. Passengers were starting to collect their belongings and tidy up their sleeping bags. No one was moving to the exits, though, and I soon learned why. Apparently, whenever it was below zero, the temperature inside the ferry had to equal that outside. It had something to do with the fact that the vessel was old. The silence following the cutting of the engines simply indicated a period of waiting for it to get colder.

Those people were right. If I get off this boat alive, it truly will be a miracle, I thought, although Marina and her mother were staying close and doing their best to nurse me and keep me warm. How lucky I was to have the attention of such good people. Without them, I guessed my chances would be close to zero.

After what seemed an eternity, the hatch was slowly opened. A freezing fog drifted around the opening as everyone started to move towards the exit. My guardian angels, as

I thought of them, called on Chief Running Water for his assistance. Without hesitation, he sent over two of his sons. They were strapping young men, well built, and over six-feet tall. They laid out what appeared to be a huge bearskin, asked me to lie on it, and proceeded to lift me up and carry me off the ferry. The next thing I remembered was waking up to find myself in a warmly furnished cabin with Marina standing over me.

"Your fever broke last night," she said. "After what you have experienced, you are very lucky to be alive. We were not sure we could save you, but some higher being had dictated that you would live. We have seen a miracle. Everybody says it's a miracle."

With some difficulty, I raised my head and enquired as to how long I had been there. "Three days," was her reply, "but don't let that worry you. We have to get you well before you can think of doing anything else."

Reassured and feeling comfortable and warm, I watched the flicker of firelight reflecting off the exposed roof beams. I fell into another deep sleep.

The next thing I knew, someone was looking down at me. This time it was not Marina, but Sylvia. When she saw me opening my eyes and noticed I was regaining some colour in my cheeks, the sadness in her blue eyes changed to a look of relief and then happiness. She knew what that meant.

I was in my room in Intensive Care, and how I had been transported back from across the lake, I will never know. The important thing was I had beaten the pneumonia.

Author Acknowledgements

Grateful thanks to my wife, Sylvia, for her help and patience. I also want to acknowledge and thank: Brian Taylor and the team at Pneuma Books, for a superb job; Sarah Campbell, at Trafford, for her help and support; and Carol Richard, for her assistance in proof-reading.

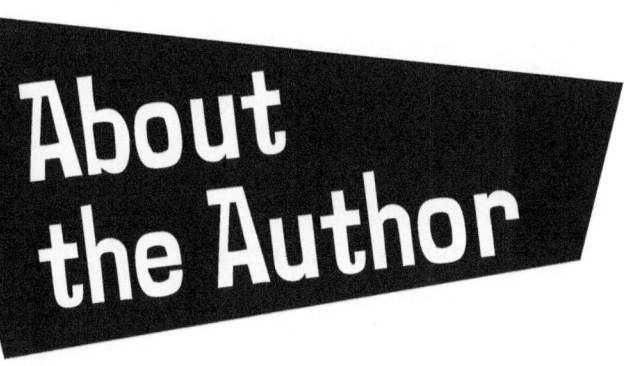

About the Author

Brian was born in Derbyshire, England in 1928. He was educated at the West Bridgford Grammar School, Nottingham. After two years of service in the British Army, he embarked on an accounting career, which eventually led to a senior financial position in Salisbury, Wiltshire. In 1977, having achieved his career ambition, he emigrated for the second time, to the 'Blue Sky country' — Alberta, Canada — with his wife and three daughters, seeking new challenges.

It was in June 1998 when he met with a catastrophic life-threatening illness, Guillain-Barré Syndrome. At the time of his frightening encounter with that disease, Brian was a healthy 'young' sixty-nine year old International Sales Manager. He was an enthusiastic golfer, even if, in his own words, not particularly good. In addition, he enjoyed various other hobbies, each one calling in its own way for physical fitness. These included gardening, model railroading, and walking.

He had, and still has, a keen interest in nature. He loved to spend much of his leisure time walking and enjoying the wildlife that was so abundant in the area close to his home in Calgary.

His first book, A First Step — Understanding Guillain-Barré Syndrome, was a personal account of a battle for survival against a severe, acute, chronic, axonal form of that rare disease, and his subsequent determination to return to as normal a life as possible. His story should be an inspiration to others.

Brian S. Langton first hit upon the idea of writing that book while lying, virtually paralysed, in a rehabilitation ward. He had earlier been stricken with a particularly serious form of Guillain-Barré Syndrome, sometimes referred to as G.B.S., and had already spent over seven months in intensive care, more than six of those months on a ventilator for breathing assistance. He had recovered his ability to speak, and was becoming used to entertaining visitors by recounting some of the dream sequences he had experienced during his period of hospitalisation. He was interested and encouraged by the positive messages he appeared to be providing to his visitors. Many of the dreams were quite hilarious, in spite of Brian's serious predicament, and it occurred to him that a collection of them would make for interesting reading. It had also become evident that few had experience of G.B.S., and he was constantly being made aware of just how rare the illness was, and of the nursing community's appetite for knowledge about the

168

About the Author

Syndrome. It was this realization which prompted Brian to seriously consider writing a book, not just about the dream sequences but to produce a sort of hand-book on G.B.S., suitable for medical professionals, caregivers, G.B.S. patients and relatives, alike.

Upon eventual discharge from hospital, Brian carried these thoughts home. He could not write at that time. It was only just possible for him to move his right arm in a limited way from the shoulder. His recreational therapist had arranged a one-finger splint to allow him to use a computer keyboard by pressing one key at a time, but it would take more than that to write a book, or so he thought. It was not until a student caregiver convinced him that he was physically capable of writing the book he was contemplating, even if it meant using 'voice software' and possibly, if the worst came to the worst, by the one finger typing method.

Thus encouraged, and in spite of no writing experience, Brian, with the help and encouragement of that student, commenced work on his book at the start of the new millennium, January 2000.

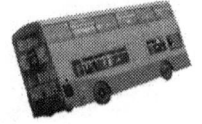